I Have Diabetes, What Next?

Preventing and managing the spectrum of metabolic dysfunction ranging from Prediabetes to Metabolic Syndrome

Table of Contents

Raw Revolution, LLC
46 Oxford Road
New Hartford, NY 13413
1-11150686811

ISBN 978-1-7326757-0-4 (ebook)
ISBN 978-1-7326757-1-1 (paperback)

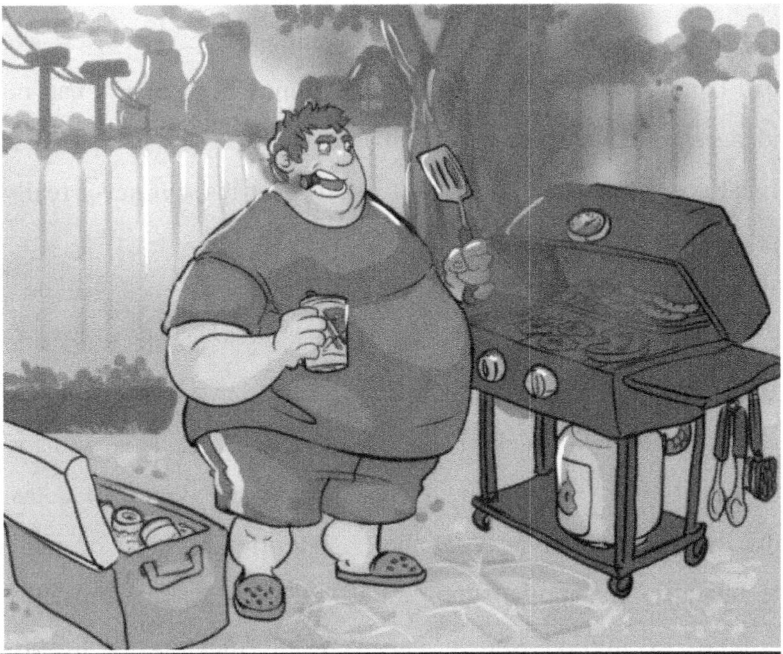

INTRODUCTION

A few years ago, as I approached my late 40's, I started experiencing frequent aches and pains. I had back pain, stiff joints, problems sleeping, and I was getting forgetful. My muscles got squishy. I woke up in the middle of the night with leg cramps. Soon after, I noticed problems with urination and there was constant dry mouth and thirst. I initially chalked it all up to old age and like many, I put off going to the doctor. I knew the doctor would scold me for being overweight and for not exercising. One day, my family was gathered at my parent's house, and my physician sister took one look at me and forced me to test my blood sugar using a simple finger prick test she had handy for my elderly parents. Up until that point, I had no idea such a device was even available, or how easy it was to use. I had seen the ads on cable TV for testing strips, but never really paid much attention.

My blood sugar was over 250. I had no idea that this, according to my sister, was "off the charts". My sister started to scold me, saying that I was very likely to have a stroke in the next year or two unless I changed my lifestyle. This was my introduction to what we call pre-diabetes, behavioral diabetes, diabetes mellitus, type 2 Diabetes, late-life diabetes, or more technically, metabolic syndrome (MetS). There are presently around 30 million known card-carrying members with this disease in the United States. Every year, we add one and a half million more. By 2050, it is estimated that one out of every three American adults will have diabetes.[1] For people over sixty-five, estimates claim eight out of ten have diabetes.[2]

Diabetes is deadly because it is generally silent. Because the deterioration caused by diabetes is slow, things like cramps, nerve pain, gout, waves of arthritic bone pain, loss of your hearing and eyesight, paralysis, or dementia will not happen overnight. Every year or two, something new stops working the way it should. Most people that suffer from behavioral late-life diabetes don't realize they have this constant severe level of metabolic dysfunction until they experience a catastrophic event like a stroke, break brittle bones like their hip or ribs after a common fall, or begin to have noticeable dementia symptoms.[3] Like I did, many blame the subtle changes to eyesight, new pains and aches, and stiffer joints to "aging", which is partially true.[4] Aging can certainly contribute to disease. Diabetes, however, can accelerate aging exponentially.

Even before there were blood tests that could quantify blood glucose and cholesterol, apothecaries throughout history looked for the "honey urine" that attracted ants, gout, and gangrene. The ancients knew that the cause of this late-life condition was rich food, alcohol, and tobacco, and the condition was referred to as the *disease of kings* because rich food, alcohol, and tobacco were readily available to people in power.[5]

Times have changed. Rich food, alcohol, and tobacco are readily available to everyone these days. As more people indulge in a Western lifestyle, the medical and scientific community started to see an explosion of the symptoms of diabetes. These days, if you're moderately obese (waist/pant size in men of around 40 or women around 24), you use alcohol intermittently and maybe smoke, you will need to start to make several lifestyle changes after the age of fifty.

A major misconception is that people think that the cause of diabetes is too much sugar in the blood. But oily fat intake, and not sugar is actually the main cause of diabetes. In later stages of the disease, when the pancreas stops producing enough insulin resulting in ineffective blood sugar management, high blood sugar levels become a major concern, but in most cases, fixing behavioral diabetes has little to do with average sugar intake levels unless your pancreas is malfunctioning.

Doctors have now developed standards based on blood tests and vital signs to catch the silent creep of diabetes mellitus before obvious signs surface like gout or gangrene. These days, doctors diagnose diabetes mellitus when a cluster of abnormal results occur together. When you go for a check-up, your doctor will measure how much fat, cholesterol, and sugar is free-flowing around in your blood, how long your blood sugar has been erratically spiking (glycated hemoglobin, HbA1c, or A1c), whether your blood vessels are restricted (blood pressure), how much oxygen saturates your extremities, and how hard your heart is working (pulse). When several of these results are abnormal, your doctor will diagnose you with diabetes or Metabolic Syndrome (MetS). The good news is that science has advanced so much that you can now perform most of these tests in the convenience of your home. Don't get nervous, you will learn in much greater detail how to monitor all these gauges in Chapter 1 and the cause of diabetes in Chapter 2.

Just like it happened with me, when test results show abnormal results, your doctor will tell you that you have diabetes/metabolic syndrome (MetS).[6] When I was given this news, I went from book to book looking for answers. Different supposed "experts" suggested different types of diets, where they would pick on one of the three major macronutrients (carbohydrate, fat, or protein) and proclaim it the enemy. I read about the South Beach, Atkins/Keto, Mediterranean, vegetarian, vegan, smoothie, juice, and other diets. These voices were telling me to starve myself, become an athlete, or stuff myself with meat.

I quickly realized these fad diets are all gibberish. First, these diets are not sustainable for long enough to be able to eliminate the cluster of conditions that make up diabetes mellitus. Also, meat diets starve you of carbohydrates and fill you up with meat and fat, giving you bad breath, diarrhea, headaches, backaches, and cramps, while spiking cholesterol levels. I also looked at a bunch of cookbooks supposedly designed for diabetics, but as I learned more about the science, I realized these cookbooks were just as flawed because the focus was still on the glycemic index (sugar content). Glycemic control for a diabetic is like putting a band-aid on a wound that needs stitches. It probably is not enough, and in the rare case that it is, it will take a very long time to heal.

After a lot of reading, it became clear to me that the constellation of conditions they call diabetes mellitus was really all about how "swampy" conditions develop inside our bodies causing a slowdown of metabolism and increase in inflammation. The swamp prevents proper energy management which eventually causes the accumulation of sugar in the blood. This swamp is the direct consequence of a lifetime of consumption of an animal-based, fried, ultra-processed, fatty, creamy diet laced with chemicals and toxins. Sugar only becomes a problem after waxy fats and spent proteins accumulate in the circulatory and muscular system.[7] The resulting metabolic slowdown is compounded over time and starts to damage internal organs.[8] Once organs involved in metabolism, like the liver, kidneys, and pancreas are weakened, the swampy condition inside you will coat and block insulin receptors to the point where highly processed sugars start to erratically spike your blood sugar levels.[9]

Now, before we get started, let me give you a caveat. Throughout this book I will use words like thicken, milky, greasy, waxy, clog, crystallize, gunk, sandpaper, calcify, swamp, and so on, and these terms are intended to be visual aids. Organic processes are complicated and involve many different and varied factors. My goal here is to explain metabolic slowdown without using scientific terms. Also, every statement of fact in this book is supported by a citation. Sometimes animal studies are used to support a claim and other times human studies. For our purposes, animals follow the same general laws of biology. We share a great deal of our DNA blueprint with furry little mice. We can feed a mouse a Western-style diet, watch it plump up, observe how high the animal's blood pressure goes, and see whether it has a heart attack. Since we are not using animal studies to tease out damage to functions like speech or cognition, which are exclusively human, animal studies are pretty good predictors of what a Western diet can do to us humans. So, although not all the citations are from human-based studies, know that all the recommendations in this book are based on the best scientific evidence I could find.

One additional major obstacle that makes it more difficult to manage diabetes is a lack of healthcare. As I mentioned, you can go about with your life for years with daily blood pressure spikes, abnormal cholesterol, and high blood sugar, and not know it. In fact, many Americans don't get any real healthcare before Medicare kicks in at the age of sixty-five. For those under the age of sixty-five who do have good healthcare and are fortunate enough to visit their doctor on an annual basis, doctors will warn of pre-diabetes when any blood work or vitals are out of the normal range, but the American medical system is not then designed to provide preventative or holistic care. Doctors are trained to practice medicine and treat a variety of vascular, circulatory, and digestive disorders, diseases, and cancers that are a consequence of diabetes mellitus. They are not trained to be nutritionists and counselors who can help someone naturally reverse the cluster of conditions that cause the metabolic slowdown that leads to diabetes mellitus and eventually metabolic syndrome.

That's what I do in this book. I walk you through step-by-step and show you how to diagnose and reverse diabetes. Knowledge is power. If you wait too long, the damage will be too great to repair. To me, sleeping through the night and the freedom from pain that came about from changing my lifestyle was enough incentive. For others, it may be the ability to work longer, live longer, avoid dementia, stop the suffering, or to slow down the progression of disease.

If you don't want to make some rather simple lifestyle changes, or if your life *still* revolves around the pleasure you get from a Western diet and lifestyle, this is probably not the book for you. There is an old saying: You can lead the horse to water, but you can't make it drink.

---

[1]https://www.cdc.gov/media/pressrel/2010/r101022.html

[2]Chentli F, Azzoug S, Mahgoun S. Diabetes mellitus in elderly. *Indian Journal of Endocrinology and Metabolism.* 2015;19(6):744-752. doi:10.4103/2230-8210.167553.

[3] Khan RMM, Chua ZJY, Tan JC, Yang Y, Liao Z, Zhao Y. From Pre-Diabetes to Diabetes: Diagnosis, Treatments and Translational Research. *Medicina (Kaunas).* 2019;55(9):546. Published 2019 Aug 29. doi:10.3390/medicina55090546

[4] Stallone G, Infante B, Prisciandaro C, Grandaliano G. mTOR and Aging: An Old Fashioned Dress. *Int J Mol Sci.* 2019;20(11):2774. Published 2019 Jun 6. doi:10.3390/ijms20112774

[5] Lakhtakia R. The history of diabetes mellitus. *Sultan Qaboos Univ Med J.* 2013;13(3):368–370.

Nuki G, Simkin PA. A concise history of gout and hyperuricemia and their treatment. *Arthritis Res Ther.* 2006;8 Suppl 1(Suppl 1):S1. doi:10.1186/ar1906

Sanders LJ. From Thebes to Toronto and the 21st century: An incredible journey. Diabetes Spectrum. 2002;15:56–60. doi: 10.2337/diaspect.15.1.56.

[6] Parikh RM, Mohan V. Changing definitions of metabolic syndrome. *Indian J Endocrinol Metab.* 2012;16(1):7-12. doi:10.4103/2230-8210.91175

[7] Bhowmik B, Siddiquee T, Mujumder A, et al. Serum Lipid Profile and Its Association with Diabetes and Prediabetes in a Rural Bangladeshi

Population. *Int J Environ Res Public Health.* 2018;15(9):1944. Published 2018 Sep 6. doi:10.3390/ijerph15091944

[8] Sargis RM, Howard SG, Newbold RR, Heindel JJ. THE DIABETES EPIDEMIC: Environmental Chemical Exposure in Etiology and Treatment. *San Franc Med.* 2012;85(5):18-20.

[9] Ramteke P, Deb A, Shepal V, Bhat MK. Hyperglycemia Associated Metabolic and Molecular Alterations in Cancer Risk, Progression, Treatment, and Mortality. *Cancers (Basel).* 2019;11(9):1402. Published 2019 Sep 19. doi:10.3390/cancers11091402

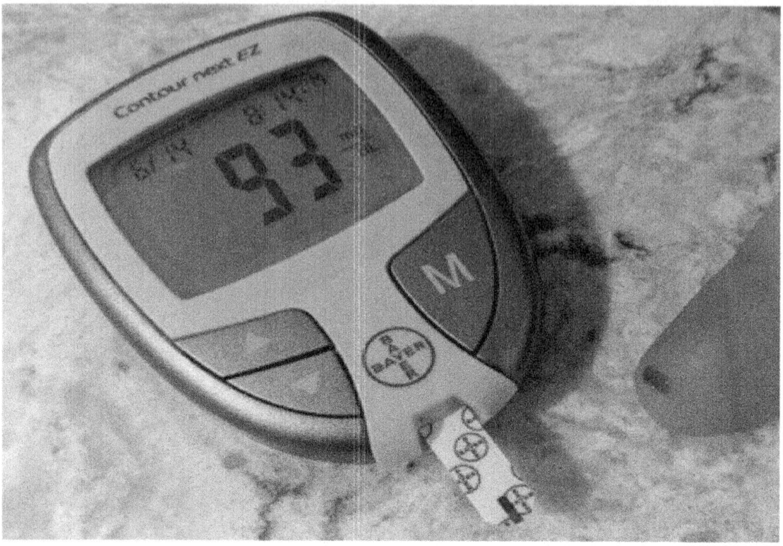

CHAPTER 1

KNOWLEDGE IS POWER

How do you know if something is wrong? There is no single clear set of symptoms for metabolic dysfunction. This uncertainty is why diabetes mellitus is called the silent killer. To catch this silent disease as early as possible, the medical and scientific community has developed very simple tests from which you can determine how bad things are. You can measure how much fat, cholesterol, and sugar is free-flowing around in your blood, how much sugar coats your red blood cells (glycated hemoglobin, HbA1c, or A1c), whether your blood vessels are restricted (blood pressure), how much oxygen is flowing around in your extremities (oxygen saturation), and how hard your heart is working (pulse). Doctors use these blood tests and vital signs to diagnose Metabolic Syndrome or MetS. The marketplace has also made several advances, allowing for us to check these levels right from home. The home tests are reasonably priced and sufficiently accurate.

CHOLESTEROL AND TRIGLYCERIDE MONITOR

I recently was in arbitration with a high-level retired judge. As we were waiting for the insurance company to painfully muster up an unreasonable offer of settlement, he explained to me how he was sitting on the bench one day, when suddenly he became so physically ill that an ambulance had to be summoned. At the hospital, he was told that he had blood leakage around his heart that almost ended his life. This judge was not by any means overweight in my visual estimation. He then proceeded to tell me how for decades his favorite once or twice a day meal was fast food combos (processed meat, fried potatoes, and a sugary drink).

A major cause of late-life diabetes and the complications it brings about, like blood leakage around the heart, is high fat (triglyceride) and high cholesterol blood levels. Over time, this build-up causes inflammation, stiffens blood pathways, creates plaque, and causes lesions.[10] Oils and fats gone unused will thicken, congeal, solidify, and eventually calcify inside you. Blood pathways will lose their rigidity and cause leaks or clog. A lifetime of high triglyceride and cholesterol blood levels will also very likely result in some form of late-life diabetes because fat and cholesterol accumulation blocks insulin signals. As we age, we have a harder time cleaning and clearing out the greasy and waxy fats we eat.[11] Excess fat in our blood settles on cells and prevents insulin from signaling cells to burn energy. Cholesterol turns into foamy fats that eventually turn into plaques in and around our heart, liver, major arteries, and brain.[12]

We can monitor triglyceride (TG) and total cholesterol (TC) blood levels right from home. There is a simple and easy-to-use home test to measure your blood triglyceride (TG) and total cholesterol (TC) levels. You insert the right test chip and correct test strip into the testing machine, prick a finger, draw enough blood to saturate the test strip, and the device will display the result in a few seconds. The total cholesterol (TC) and triglyceride (TG) test is affordable ($1.50 per test strip for a total of $3.00) and relatively accurate given that it is a finger prick test. The best time to check TG and TC levels is after an overnight fast. Do the test every morning for three days in a row. If every single day you are over the numbers of 200 (TG) and 240 (TC), you eat too much meaty, fried, oily, fatty, creamy food. Although you may have heard that different densities of cholesterol (high (HDL) low (LDL) and very low-density lipoproteins (VLDL) can be categorized as good and bad cholesterol, these variations are not important to us. Your doctor can monitor those for you. We only care about total cholesterol and triglyceride blood levels.

A diet high in ground fatty meats and/or foods fried in oil will spike blood triglyceride levels above the acceptable limit of 200 mg/dL, and gradually increase blood cholesterol levels above 240 mg/dL.[13] I'm sure you have heard people refer to a creamy, meaty, fatty, fried meal as a heart attack on a plate, or make comments after such a meal that they can feel their arteries stiffening? These claims are not exactly true, but a sustained diet, year after year, high in animal products and oil will eventually overload your body so that pockets of congealed or calcified gunk start to accumulate inside you, preventing the processing of sugar in your body. The only defense your body has is to burn this gunk away or break it down by attacking it which results in inflammation. Your body will do the best it can to clean and clear, but you can seriously help it along if you stop eating foods that are fried and oily and if you start a regiment of exercise to combat a sedentary state during aging.

The diet in this book offers a very effective way to reduce blood triglyceride (TG) and cholesterol (TC) levels in four months. The diet offered acts as a wash cycle to clean your blood of triglyceride and cholesterol. While on the diet, you should test triglyceride (TG) and total cholesterol (TC) levels once or twice a week until the downward curve starts to flatten, and then test once or twice a month. Make a chart so you can write down the results and compare them.

BLOOD SUGAR MONITOR

If you eat too much sweet chocolate and sugary candies, your pancreas and liver will convert the excess unused digestible sugars into energy and eventually fat.[14] The unused excess can get stored as fat in the liver, leading to a fatty liver, or stored in fat cells throughout the body, leading to weight gain. So, sugar can also contribute secondarily to diabetes if consumed in high quantities.

After years of bad eating, the body stores and accumulates fatty pockets. These fatty pockets come in different sizes and shapes. The fat can accumulate in your muscles, giving it that marbled look, or grow in between your arterial skin, causing blockage, or accumulate in major organs, causing inflammation or malfunction. This accumulation magnifies the effect of insulin resistance as we age, so it is common to hear experts recommend glycemic control as blood sugar management starts to become a constant daily struggle, especially in elderly diabetics.

If you are past the age of fifty and you have eaten an exclusively Western diet all your life, you may notice that when you eat a chocolate-covered gooey, yummy candy bar, and test your blood sugar a couple of hours later, there will be an abnormal spike in blood sugar levels, and for many of you, it can take several hours for your blood sugar levels to return to normal. As the years go by, the duration of these blood sugar spikes will increase even as you consume smaller doses of these processed sugar foods. Eventually, it will get to a point where a couple of slices of white bread, relatively moderate in sugar and carbohydrates, will start to spike blood sugar levels for six or more hours. When the blood is saturated with excess sugar for several hours a day, you will start to notice a high A1c level (next section), which is where the sugar starts to settle on your red blood cells, causing even more noticeable metabolic dysfunction.

Just like blood fat levels, we can monitor blood sugar levels right from home. Using test strips inserted into a device with a drop of blood, you can find out your blood sugar (glucose) level. To determine how good your body is doing in clearing sugar out of your blood, fast overnight starting at around 6 pm, then take your baseline blood sugar level in the morning before you eat anything around 8 am. Follow this with a hearty Western-style processed meal (fried food, flour, sugary drink, and a chocolate dessert) and take your blood sugar level two hours later, and again four hours after your meal. There should be a bell curve (∩). Your blood sugar should be 85-95mg/dL (~5mmol/L) right before you start eating for the day after an overnight fast, and no more than 140mg/dL (~8mmol/L) after a meal.

For diabetics, this bell curve is much wider. If your fasting blood sugar level (baseline) refuses to get to 95mg/dL (~5mmol/L) and instead stays stubbornly at 130mg/dL (~7mmol/L) or more after your fast, if your blood sugar level two hours after a meal still remains above 180mg/dL

(~10mmol/L), or if your blood sugar remains high at 130 to 180mg/dL (~7-10mmol/L) four or six hours after you eat, this means that you are very likely a diabetic and that you have had blood sugar management issues for a while.

The Wash Cycle Diet in this book will optimize your blood sugar levels within a few days. Once optimized, you need only monitor your blood sugar in the morning a couple of times a week. Once you have finished the Washing Cycle, and if you decide to add more western or processed foods back into your diet, you should test the effects using the same staggered testing: fast, 2-hour and 4-hour, to make sure you are not returning to a state of insulin resistance.

GLYCATED HEMOGLOBIN (A1C/HBA1C) TEST

Uncontrolled long term high blood sugar levels will cause that excess sugar to settle on red blood cells, start to harden like sandpaper, and cause inflammation.[15] A high A1c level will confirm that you have been suffering from high blood triglyceride, cholesterol, and sugar levels for a while.

At a recent court conference, I met an attorney I have done many battles with over the years. He lives in a more rural area and was an active snowmobiler, hunter, and fisher. He was in his late sixties and did not abuse alcohol or smoke. He was having a tough time keeping his A1c levels from rising. He told me that he was never a sugarholic, but that he really enjoyed fried food, particularly fried onion rings. Even though he was not a big fan of sweets, fat from years of eating fried food, even despite his constant movement, was creating enough insulin resistance to raise his A1c level.

A1c can also be easily tested at home without a prescription. The A1c test is similar in application to the triglyceride, total cholesterol, and blood glucose tests. You saturate a strip with blood, insert it into a small device, and get the result. You only need to perform an A1C test once a month. An optimal A1c level is just below 5%.[16] If your number is above 6%, most doctors would consider you pre-diabetic, and at 7% fully diabetic.[17] If your A1c is over 7%, you probably have Metabolic Syndrome (MetS).

The only way to get rid of a high A1c level (glycated hemoglobin) is to replace your red blood cells in a clean environment. Red blood cells have a life span of about four months, and these cells are constantly dying and being replaced. So, if you take the test about once a month, you will detect any noticeable changes in your A1c levels. This is also why the Wash Cycle Diet duration offered in this book is set at four months. If your A1c level is high, after following the diet for four months, you will get back to an optimal A1c level.

To recap, blood sugar levels get erratic after a sustained diet high in fat and cholesterol. Diets high in processed sugar also contribute to a lesser degree to the increase in insulin resistance. The longer blood sugar levels remain erratic, the higher your A1C level. You can manage your blood sugar levels with glycemic control, but unless you reduce or eliminate the consumption of cholesterol, oil, and frying, you will slowly get worse. If you fail to manage your blood sugar and you keep eating fried animal products, you will experience gout, squishy muscles, brittle bones, deteriorated eyesight and hearing, and eventually even diabetic gangrene.

Pulse Oximeter

Life depends on oxygen. Oxygen is a major component of energy units made by the cells called ATP (Adenosine Triphosphate). When any part of the body is even momentarily deprived of oxygen, bad things happen.[18] Low blood oxygen saturation levels, especially in the outer extremities, significantly accelerate organ and nervous system damage through two processes: oxidative stress,[19] and inflammation.[20] When your body gets so clogged that the blood delivering oxygen starts to have trouble getting to your extremities, you need to reverse course immediately.

A pulse oximeter tests low oxygen saturation levels in the extremities. A pulse oximeter can instantly determine oxygen saturation levels by placement over the finger or toe and does not require any pricking or pain. Simply place the device over a finger or a toe, wait a few seconds, and the device will measure wavelengths to see how well oxygen is getting saturated in the furthest points of the body. An optimal oxygen saturation level in the extremities is 99%. If you remain healthy as you age, your oxygen saturation levels should always remain above 96%, and preferably as high as 98% or 99%. When levels start to drop to 94%, you will have serious metabolic dysfunction. If oxygen saturation levels are consistently below 92%, you should immediately talk to a doctor. If you have oxygen saturation levels below 89%, many doctors will prescribe oxygen therapy (the use of an oxygen concentrator through tubes in your nose).

My mother recently broke her hip at the age of eighty-five. Immediately after the surgery, her blood oxygen saturation levels dropped to 85%. As she lay immobile in the hospital bed, I noticed that she had significant trouble catching her breath. X-rays of her lungs started to show major obstruction and we thought she was destined to pass away. I started encouraging her to sit up and I would lightly stretch her for an hour during daily visits while using a vibrating massager all over her lower body. Eventually, I was able to get her to stand using a walker. Within a couple of weeks, along with the help of medication, she was able to significantly increase the blood oxygen saturation levels in her extremities.

Therefore, it is important to check your oxygen saturation levels every day. Even the slightest slowdown or interference with metabolism will immediately become apparent with an oximeter.[21] Most pre-diabetic or type 2 diabetics have a stubbornly borderline oxygen saturation level of 96% or less, which is still at the bottom of the normal range. Even this borderline oxygen saturation level is an indicator that bad things are happening inside.

If you are already have low blood oxygen levels, you probably also have sleep disturbance like apnea (where you stop breathing for short periods during sleep).[22] If you have insomnia,[23] wake up more than occasionally with a headache after a full night's sleep,[24] your significant other reports that you snore,[25] or if you take several cat naps during the day,[26] you should report such things to your doctor. Many obese aging diabetics have sleep apnea.[27] If you detect the problem early enough, you can get a prescription from your doctor for a CPAP (Continuous Positive Airway Pressure) machine to help level pressure in your airways as you sleep. A CPAP machine prevents the muscles in your throat from collapsing during sleep while feeding air into the lungs. An oxygen concentrator and CPAP machine are wonderful tools that can extend the life of diabetics for many years.[28]

BLOOD PRESSURE MONITOR

The ancients used to describe high blood pressure through symptoms like tense veins or fullness of pulse, burning feet, or a foggy mind which usually resulted in rapid loss of eyesight.[29] By the time these symptoms became apparent, however, you were likely just a skip away from a life-threatening stroke. Today, we have blood pressure monitors that will pre-warn you years in advance. Most people who have high blood pressure are completely unaware of the condition that is slowly killing their most delicate of cells and nerves. You should start checking your blood pressure every day after the age of fifty.

Circulation, measured by oxygen saturation, blood pressure, and pulse are all part of an interrelated respiratory-circulatory-metabolic system, and the moment metabolism starts to act erratically, the result is the cluster of abnormal gauges we previously talked about, which will lead to circulation problems, tested by low oxygen saturation, high blood pressure, and high pulse rates. Usually, you also see outward signs like sleep apnea, numbness, joint pain, twitches, a foggy mind, and loss of vision or hearing. This means that the engine inside you is spitting and knocking.

A blood pressure monitor measures systolic (during pumping) and diastolic (between pumps) pressure. These numbers are reported as systolic over diastolic. The upper edge of normal when it comes to blood pressure is 120 (systolic) over 80 (diastolic) (120/80 mm Hg). If you are over forty and your systolic blood pressure is over 130, or your diastolic pressure is above 85, your pressure is elevated. If your pressure is even moderately higher,[30] your doctor may classify you as having stage one or two hypertension.

Unlike blood tests, there is no specific time of day requirement to check your blood pressure. In fact, your blood pressure will fluctuate during the day. It will be at its lowest when you wake up and before you go to bed. When you take your blood pressure, make sure you don't have a full bladder, that you didn't just drink a large caffeine drink, and wait a while if you just finished an exercise routine. I would suggest taking your blood pressure three times during the day: in the morning, in the afternoon, and before you go to bed. Record the results on a chart and look to see if there is any trend. Your evening and morning blood pressure should be about the same, and your afternoon blood pressure should be the highest. If you have lower blood pressure in the evening, but your blood pressure spikes in the morning, this is a good indication of bad sleeping patterns.[31] A high waking blood pressure usually means that you are well on your way to heart disease or a stroke.[32]

Most experts will tell you that high blood pressure or hypertension is caused by multiple factors ranging from genetics to obesity. The major causes of high blood pressure in elderly diabetics are as follows:

► obesity, especially morbid obesity.[33] The greatest reducer of blood pressure in obese people is weight loss. A loss of twenty pounds of weight can bring blood pressure down as effectively as any prescription drug on the market today. But what if you really don't have twenty pounds to lose and still suffer from high blood pressure?

► A second major cause of high blood pressure is fried foods and ground animal products.[34] Raw, boiled, or oven-cooked fish will generally have a lesser adverse effect. Experts blame Maillard Reaction Products like advanced glycoxidation end-products (AGEs) and heterocyclic amines (HCAs), which are basically burnt carbons (the black stuff on a grilled steak or hamburger), or more accurately, complex reactions of chemicals that occur when meat is ground and cooked. Other experts blame trimethylamine-N-oxide (TMAO), which is a derivative made in the liver from animal products, and which causes blood pathway rigidity and blockage, inflammation, and stress.[35] Regardless of why processed meats raise blood pressure as we age, we know it does. A recent study found that the laziest of vegans have a lower blood pressure than the most active, athletic carnivores who indulge in a Western diet.[36]

► Finally, a dose-response relationship exists between alcohol consumption and high blood pressure.[37] There is a 1 point (mm Hg) increase in blood pressure for every beer or mixed drink you consume, and it can take up to two weeks of abstinence to reverse the blood pressure spike.[38]

High blood pressure or hypertension can also mean that you are starting to develop chronic kidney disease (CKD) and a fatty liver (NAFLD). In fact, virtually every single person who has kidney disease also has high blood pressure.[39] As we age, we naturally lose kidney function, but animal studies have shown that rats with kidney disease that are fed a protein-restricted diet can still live prolonged lives. More recent human studies are also starting to show the same.[40] People with hypertension also usually have a fatty liver. Although the liver is far more regenerative than the kidneys, persistent high blood pressure often means you are developing what they call Non-Alcoholic Fatty Liver Disease (NAFLD).[41]

High blood pressure will cause damage to cells, nerves, systems, and eventually to organs in your body. Chronic high blood pressure can accelerate the onset of blindness, stroke, and heart failure. Life insurance companies look critically at your blood pressure levels and whether you are taking any medication to bring down your blood pressure when deciding whether to offer you protection. Disability insurance companies are even more cautious and will usually not offer good disability insurance to people who suffer from high blood pressure.

Peripheral Blood Pressure

Another important gauge to monitor regularly is your peripheral blood pressure. This is the pressure in your ankles. The ratio between your ankle blood pressure and arm blood pressure is a good indicator of whether you're suffering from peripheral artery disease.[42] You can measure peripheral blood pressure by wrapping the monitor around the ankle for measurement. Your ankle blood pressure should be higher than your arm blood pressure.[43]

If the blood pressure in your arm is higher than the blood pressure in your ankle, you should consult a doctor immediately. This means that you have peripheral artery disease and that you are much more likely to have major complications and die. There are also some physical manifestations that are giveaways like a blackened tint around the eyes, fingertips, or toes, especially when exposed to cold weather.[44] A while back, I had a deposition in the middle of winter at a prison in upstate New York. My adversary and I had to endure the cold outdoors for about twenty minutes before we were buzzed in. He was a tall gentleman and not obese, and he was not wearing gloves or a hat. Once we settled inside, I noticed that he had a dark tint around his eyes and fingertips. This tinting is a major sign of peripheral artery disease. This attorney is no longer with us.

PULSE

The final important vital is your pulse, which is timed over a period of one minute and indicates how hard your heart is working while at rest. An oximeter or a blood pressure monitor will also provide your pulse rate. Resting pulse goes up when your heart is forced to work harder to keep everything balanced. People with high resting heart rates are usually pre-diabetic or diabetic.[45] Resting heart rates can range from 50 to 100 beats per minute (bpm), and the lower the heart rate, the more efficient your circulatory/cardiovascular system is working. Every ten beats per minute increase in resting heart rate decrease your life span by 8% to 9%. Those with a resting heart rate in the eighties and nineties are at a "significantly increased risk of cardiovascular mortality".[46] Weight loss,[47] exercise or yoga,[48] are all great ways to lower standing pulse rates.[49]

FINAL NOTES

By following the recommendations in this book, you will see significant improvement in your metabolic health. In a recent study, people were put on four days of bed rest and given either a normal hospital diet or a bean diet consisting of lentils, beans, chickpeas, and peas. Insulin resistance, bone resorption, and cardiovascular factors all improved with the bean diet.[50] The stricter you are with the Wash Cycle diet in this book, the more weight you will lose (up to 20% of your body weight). Once the Wash Cycle Diet normalizes triglyceride (TG), total cholesterol (TC), blood glucose, and A1c levels for a sustained period,[51] 30 minutes of daily walking will optimize your oxygen saturation levels, blood pressure and pulse.

To summarize, the tools you need are a blood pressure monitor, an oximeter, a prick, testing strips, a reader for A1c, glucose, total cholesterol, and triglycerides. The following chart is a quick reference guide that covers all the blood levels/vitals that we discussed.

Total Cholesterol (TC)	<200 mg/dL Optimal	200-239 mg/dL Borderline	≥240 mg/dL High
Triglycerides (TG)	<150 mg/dL Fast Level	150 to 199 mg/dL Borderline	≥200 mg/dL High
Blood Glucose	85-95 mg/dL Fast Level	100-140mg/dL 2 hours after meal	>140mg/dL High
AIC	≤5.0% Optimal	6% Bordeline	≥7% High
Blood Pressure	≤ 120 Systolic ≤80 Diastolic (mm Hg)	≤ 130 Systolic ≤85 Diastolic Stage1	≤ 140 Systolic ≤90 Diastolic Stage2

	Normal	Hypertension	Hypertension
Blood Oxygenation	>96% Optimal	89-95% Borderline	<89% Low
Resting Pulse	≤60 bpm Optimal	≤80 bpm Borderline	>90 bpm High

No one is immune from metabolic deterioration after the age of fifty. Knowledge is power. This chapter arms you with the tools that will give you knowledge about your health status. The next chapter will explain why there is a diabetes creep during aging.

---

[10] Linton MRF, Yancey PG, Davies SS, et al. The Role of Lipids and Lipoproteins in Atherosclerosis. 2019 Jan 3. In: Feingold KR, Anawalt B, Boyce A, et al., editors. Endotext [Internet]. South Dartmouth (MA): MDText.com, Inc.; 2000-.

[11] Wang M, Hou X, Hu W, Chen L, Chen S. Serum lipid and lipoprotein levels of middle-aged and elderly Chinese men and women in Shandong Province. *Lipids Health Dis*. 2019;18(1):58. Published 2019 Mar 4. doi:10.1186/s12944-019-1000-0

[12] Nam KW, Kwon HM, Jeong HY, Park JH, Kwon H, Jeong SM. High triglyceride/HDL cholesterol ratio is associated with silent brain infarcts in a healthy population. *BMC Neurol*. 2019;19(1):147. Published 2019 Jul 2. doi:10.1186/s12883-019-1373-8

[13] Cox RA, García-Palmieri MR. Cholesterol, Triglycerides, and Associated Lipoproteins. In: Walker HK, Hall WD, Hurst JW, editors. Clinical Methods: The History, Physical, and Laboratory Examinations. 3rd edition. Boston: Butterworths; 1990. Chapter 31.

[14] Duwaerts CC, Maher JJ. Macronutrients and the Adipose-Liver Axis in Obesity and Fatty Liver. *Cell Mol Gastroenterol Hepatol*. 2019;7(4):749-761. doi:10.1016/j.jcmgh.2019.02.001

[15] Liu S, Hempe JM, McCarter RJ, Li S, Fonseca VA. Association between Inflammation and Biological Variation in Hemoglobin A1c in U.S. Nondiabetic Adults. *J Clin Endocrinol Metab.* 2015;100(6):2364–2371. doi:10.1210/jc.2014-4454

[16]Saleh J. Glycated hemoglobin and its spinoffs: Cardiovascular disease markers or risk factors? *World Journal of Cardiology*. 2015;7(8):449-453. doi:10.4330/wjc.v7.i8.449.

[17]Use of Glycated Haemoglobin (HbA1c) in the Diagnosis of Diabetes Mellitus: Abbreviated Report of a WHO Consultation. Geneva: World Health Organization; 2011. 2, Glycated haemoglobin (HbA1c) for the diagnosis of diabetes. Available from: https://www.ncbi.nlm.nih.gov/books/NBK304271/

[18] Pilkauskaite G, Miliauskas S, Sakalauskas R. Reactive oxygen species production in peripheral blood neutrophils of obstructive sleep apnea patients. *ScientificWorldJournal*. 2013;2013:421763. Published 2013 May 12. doi:10.1155/2013/421763

[19] Hafen BB, Sharma S. Oxygen Saturation. [Updated 2019 Jun 2]. In: StatPearls [Internet]. Treasure Island (FL): StatPearls Publishing; 2019 Jan-.

[20] Vold ML, Aasebø U, Wilsgaard T, Melbye H. Low oxygen saturation and mortality in an adult cohort: the Tromsø study. *BMC Pulm Med.* 2015;15:9. Published 2015 Feb 12.

[21] Rambaran K, Bhagan B, Ali A, et al. High Prevalence of Diabetes Mellitus in a Cohort of Patients with Chronic Obstructive Pulmonary Disease in Trinidad, West Indies. *Turk Thorac J.* 2019;20(1):12–17. Published 2019 Jan 1. doi:10.5152/TurkThoracJ.2018.18036

[22] Kim J, Yoon DW, Lee SK, et al. Concurrent presence of inflammation and obstructive sleep apnea exacerbates the risk of metabolic syndrome: A KoGES 6-year follow-up study. *Medicine (Baltimore).* 2017;96(7):e4488. doi:10.1097/MD.0000000000004488

[23] Luyster FS, Buysse DJ, Strollo PJ Jr. Comorbid insomnia and obstructive sleep apnea: challenges for clinical practice and research. *J Clin Sleep Med.* 2010;6(2):196-204.

[24] Suzuki K, Miyamoto M, Miyamoto T, et al. Sleep apnoea headache in obstructive sleep apnoea syndrome patients presenting with morning headache:

comparison of the ICHD-2 and ICHD-3 beta criteria. *J Headache Pain.* 2015;16:56. doi:10.1186/s10194-015-0540-6

[25] Kaur S, Baslas V, Aggarwal H, Kumar P, Chand P. Snoring: an annoyance or a serious health problem (obstructive sleep apnea)?. *Indian J Community Med.* 2015;40(2):143-144. doi:10.4103/0970-0218.153889

[26] Slater G, Steier J. Excessive daytime sleepiness in sleep disorders. *J Thorac Dis.* 2012;4(6):608-616. doi:10.3978/j.issn.2072-1439.2012.10.07

[27] Wali SO, Abaalkhail B, AlQassas I, Alhejaili F, Spence DW, Pandi-Perumal SR. The correlation between oxygen saturation indices and the standard obstructive sleep apnea severity. *Ann Thorac Med.* 2020;15(2):70-75. doi:10.4103/atm.ATM_215_19

[28] Gottlieb DJ, Punjabi NM, Mehra R, et al. CPAP versus oxygen in obstructive sleep apnea. *N Engl J Med.* 2014;370(24):2276-2285. doi:10.1056/NEJMoa1306766

[29] Emtiazy M, Choopani R, Khodadoost M, Tansaz M, Dehghan S, Ghahremani Z. Avicenna's doctrine about arterial hypertension. *Acta Med Hist Adriat.* 2014;12(1):157-162.

[30] Tan JL, Thakur K. Systolic Hypertension. [Updated 2020 Jan 30]. In: StatPearls [Internet]. Treasure Island (FL): StatPearls Publishing; 2020 Jan. Available from: https://www.ncbi.nlm.nih.gov/books/NBK482472/

[31] Kishimoto A, Tochikubo O, Ohshige K. Relation between nocturnal arterial oxygen desaturation and morning blood pressure. *Clin Exp Hypertens.* 2007;29(1):51-60. doi:10.1080/10641960601096786

[32] White WB. The risk of waking-up: impact of the morning surge in blood pressure. Hypertension. 2010 Apr;55(4):835-7. doi: 10.1161/HYPERTENSIONAHA.109.148908. Epub 2010 Mar 8. PMID: 20212265; PMCID: PMC2841701.

[33] Osher E, Stern N. Obesity in elderly subjects: in sheep's clothing perhaps, but still a wolf!. *Diabetes Care.* 2009;32 Suppl 2(Suppl 2):S398-S402. doi:10.2337/dc09-S347

[34] Alexander S, Ostfeld RJ, Allen K, Williams KA. A plant-based diet and

hypertension. *J Geriatr Cardiol.* 2017;14(5):327-330. doi:10.11909/j.issn.1671-5411.2017.05.014

[35] Borgi L, Curhan GC, Willett WC, Hu FB, Satija A, Forman JP. Long-term intake of animal flesh and risk of developing hypertension in three prospective cohort studies. *J Hypertens.* 2015;33(11):2231-2238. doi:10.1097/HJH.0000000000000722

[36] Fontana L, Meyer TE, Klein S, Holloszy JO. Long-term low-calorie low-protein vegan diet and endurance exercise are associated with low cardiometabolic risk. *Rejuvenation Res.* 2007;10(2):225-234. doi:10.1089/rej.2006.0529

[37] Santana NMT, Mill JG, Velasquez-Melendez G, et al. Consumption of alcohol and blood pressure: Results of the ELSA-Brasil study. *PLoS One.* 2018;13(1):e0190239. Published 2018 Jan 8. doi:10.1371/journal.pone.0190239

[38] Puddey IB, Beilin LJ. Alcohol is bad for blood pressure. Clin Exp Pharmacol Physiol. 2006 Sep;33(9):847-52. doi: 10.1111/j.1440-1681.2006.04452.x. PMID: 16922819.

[39] Pugh D, Gallacher PJ, Dhaun N. Management of Hypertension in Chronic Kidney Disease. *Drugs.* 2019;79(4):365-379. doi:10.1007/s40265-019-1064-1

[40] Rysz J, Franczyk B, Ciałkowska-Rysz A, Gluba-Brzózka A. The Effect of Diet on the Survival of Patients with Chronic Kidney Disease. *Nutrients.* 2017;9(5):495. Published 2017 May 13. doi:10.3390/nu9050495

[41] Wang Y, Zeng Y, Lin C, Chen Z. Hypertension and non-alcoholic fatty liver disease proven by transient elastography. *Hepatol Res.* 2016;46(13):1304-1310. doi:10.1111/hepr.12688

[42]Mueller T, Hinterreiter F, Poelz W, Haltmayer M, Dieplinger B. The heart matters in diabetes: 10-Year outcomes of peripheral artery disease. *SAGE Open Medicine.* 2017;5:2050312117740988. doi:10.1177/2050312117740988.

[43]Mlačak B, Blinc A, Pohar M, Stare J. Peripheral Arterial Disease and Ankle-Brachial Pressure Index as Predictors of Mortality in Residents of Metlika County, Slovenia. *Croatian medical journal.* 2006;47(2):327-334.

[44] Wollina U, Koch A, Langner D, et al. Acrocyanosis - A Symptom with Many

Facettes. *Open Access Maced J Med Sci.* 2018;6(1):208–212. Published 2018 Jan 10. doi:10.3889/oamjms.2018.035

[45] Xu C, Zhong J, Zhu H, et al. Independent and interactive associations of heart rate and body mass index or blood pressure with type 2 diabetes mellitus incidence: A prospective cohort study. *J Diabetes Investig.* 2019;10(4):1068–1074. doi:10.1111/jdi.12999

[46] Zhang D, Shen X, Qi X. Resting heart rate and all-cause and cardiovascular mortality in the general population: a meta-analysis. *CMAJ.* 2016;188(3):E53–E63.

[47] Wasmund SL, Owan T, Yanowitz FG, et al. Improved heart rate recovery after marked weight loss induced by gastric bypass surgery: two-year follow up in the Utah Obesity Study. *Heart Rhythm.* 2011;8(1):84-90. doi:10.1016/j.hrthm.2010.10.023

[48] Reimers AK, Knapp G, Reimers CD. Effects of Exercise on the Resting Heart Rate: A Systematic Review and Meta-Analysis of Interventional Studies. *J Clin Med.* 2018;7(12):503. Published 2018 Dec 1. doi:10.3390/jcm7120503

[49] Nicoll R, Henein MY. Caloric Restriction and Its Effect on Blood Pressure, Heart Rate Variability and Arterial Stiffness and Dilatation: A Review of the Evidence. *Int J Mol Sci.* 2018;19(3):751. Published 2018 Mar 7. doi:10.3390/ijms19030751

[50] Gao R, Duff W, Chizen D, Zello GA, Chilibeck PD. The Effect of a Low Glycemic Index Pulse-Based Diet on Insulin Sensitivity, Insulin Resistance, Bone Resorption and Cardiovascular Risk Factors during Bed Rest. *Nutrients.* 2019;11(9):2012. Published 2019 Aug 27. doi:10.3390/nu11092012

[51] Wannamethee G, Shaper AG. The association between heart rate and blood pressure, blood lipids and other cardiovascular risk factors. *J Cardiovasc Risk.* 1994;1(3):223-230. doi:10.1177/174182679400100307

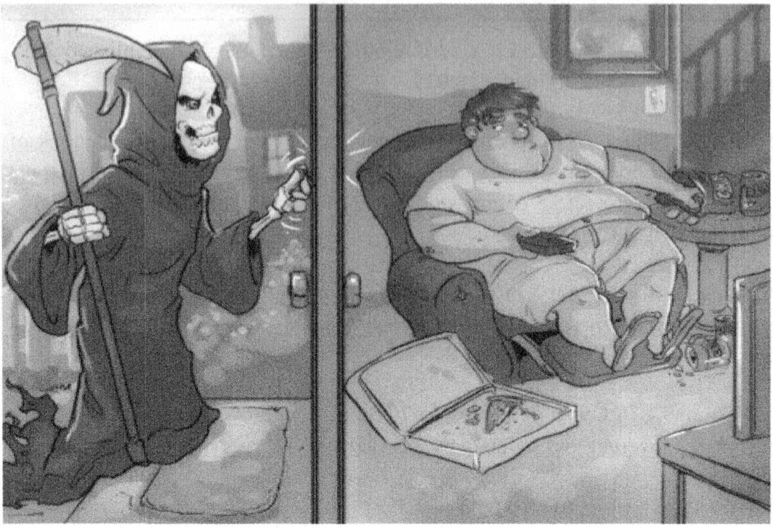

CHAPTER 2

SAD: STANDARD AMERICAN DIET

Humans have consumed alcohol, flour, milk, eggs, lard, meat, and sweets for thousands of years. Tobacco and drugs have been around for many centuries. But Western life has made these foods, alcohols, nicotine products, caffeinated drinks, and most recently marijuana products abundant, cheap, and very accessible. Convenience stores sell cigarettes, alcohol, and a variety of caffeinated drinks. Fast food restaurants serve instant, hot, processed, and delicious food at every corner, and smart entrepreneurs have figured out how to safely package many food products using freezing and preservatives.[52] You simply grab it off the shelf, throw it in a super convection rotisserie microwave oven, and shazaam, in just a short few minutes, you have great tasting state fair/hamburger joint food right in the comfort of your home.

These processed food products are highly addictive because they share characteristics with other drugs by providing rapid absorption of a high dose that induces a feeling of euphoria and satiety.[53] Oil, sugar, flour, milk products, and ground meats are highly processed, super absorbent, and highly satisfying. Because of societal advancements that allow us to feed these addictions with such abundance and so cheaply, food products, drugs, and synthetic chemicals rule Western life. Get up in the morning, you need your coffee. Three meals are recommended a day. Sugar is abundant. Until recently, cigarettes were part of the fabric of Western society. We have weekly feasts where we gather with family and friends and drink and eat to excess. Hundreds of acres of corn and wheat fields can be planted with two farmers and large industrial machines. Dairy farms can produce milk in excess amounts, and beef, pork, and chicken are cheaply mass farmed.

The consequence is that diabetes mellitus is no longer a condition reserved for the infrequent indulgent rich person that is morbidly obese.[54] As more and more people are addicted to this Western lifestyle, the devastation becomes more pronounced. One of my law school professors was an alcoholic who brought screwdrivers to class in his coffee cup. He made it to his mid-sixties. Many heavy smokers pass before their seventies.[55] There are no eighty-some-year-old morbidly obese people out there.

Indulgence in a Western diet and lifestyle drastically shortens your life span but what matters even more is the steadily decreasing quality of life that comes with indulgence.

Western Diet and Lifestyle

These days, over 90% of a Western-style diet is ultra-processed food products. We grind our meats, use oil as a main ingredient, and flour, sugar, milk, and eggs are a part of almost every meal. These food products are made from macronutrients we need to sustain life (protein, fat, and carbohydrates), except that because of ultra-processing, they are very digestible and therefore calorie-dense. These food products are the major reason we have an explosion of diabetes around the world.

Another major reason why we see an explosion of diabetes is our exposure to drugs and synthetic chemicals. Drugs have never been as accessible as they are today. We are in the midst of an opioid crisis.[56] Marijuana is now legal.[57] Alcohol, a known neurotoxin, has been around forever.[58] Nicotine, a toxic pesticide, is consumed by many people.[59] Caffeine, another known toxin, is regularly consumed.[60] According to the CDC, tens of millions of Americans use tobacco products.[61] Almost all of us drink or binge drink regularly.[62] Preservatives, perfumes, and artificially sweetened drinks have unproven safety records.[63] Chemical weapons used during World Wars such as ammonium nitrate and organophosphate nerve gas have been reinvented as fertilizers and pesticides for agriculture.[64] Six billion pounds of these pesticides are used every year,[65] and they taint virtually everything we eat. A common pesticide called glyphosate (Round-Up®) is used to increase wheat yields all over the world. Animals exposed to this herbicide develop celiac disease and cancer.[66] In humans, farmers exposed to small doses develop a particularly insidious cancer called non-Hodgkin's lymphoma.[67]

Animal meats have also become a large part of our diet and another major reason why we see an explosion of diabetes. Aside from their unhealthy protein and fat contents, farm animals are crammed into massive Concentrated Animal Feeding Operations (CAFOs),[68] given growth hormones,[69] fed enriched food,[70] exposed to industrial chemicals,[71] and carry many life-threatening pathogens.[72] Heavy antibiotic use in these facilities is creating new antibiotic-resistant superbugs and viruses capable of decimating life.[73] Anywhere from 10% to 90% of these pathogens remain active even after cooking.[74] These toxins and pathogens damage organs responsible for metabolism and accelerate the onset of diseases like Alzheimer's,[75] and Parkinson's.[76]

Because of the combination of these insults all occurring at the same time, metabolic diseases that used to pop up as often as someone winning the lottery or being struck by lightning have become regular occurrences. We especially see an explosion of nervous system disorders.[77] According to estimates, one-tenth of our population now has a significant learning or behavioral disability,[78] and emotional deficits like Aspergers, speech impediments, anxiety, and the onset of early cognitive decline are common. None of this should come as a surprise.[79] Food products, drugs, synthetic chemicals, pesticides, and pathogens are all major reasons we have an explosion of MetS and the proliferation of exotic diseases throughout the Western world.

The problem is that western food, drink, and inhaling products are designed to give us immediate pleasure.[80] A Western diet (frying, ultra-processing, cholesterol, complex proteins, and oxides), and the degree to which you indulge this Western lifestyle (overweight, stationary, indoors, THC, alcohol, nicotine, caffeine), and how protective you are to avoid pesticides and pathogens (organic, vegetarian), will determine how badly you struggle with serious metabolic disorder,[81] especially as you age.

How It Works

Ultra-processed foods are basically remnants of cells that have been highly processed and pre-treated in different ways to make oil, sugar, flour, and ground meats. Your digestive tract will absorb these ultra-pre-processed cellular remnants easily, bypassing much of the arduous processes of acid break down and fermentation that happen in the small intestine and colon, allowing warp speed passage into your bloodstream. As a result, we get that immediate and addictive feeling of euphoria and satiety. These cellular remnants come packed with dense doses of readily available energy, much of which your body really does not need unless you are an athlete or perform physical labor most of the day. But, because of how highly processed these cellular remnants are, if they are not used almost immediately, they oxidize rapidly into hard to remove and useless waxy fats and sticky proteins that are hard to break down and dissolve.

When you were young, your body did a good job of eliminating much of a Western diet that is poured into it daily. But as aging starts to slow you down, usually in your early fifties, these rapidly oxidizing cellular remnants accumulate in your body, and you start to see things like weight gain and stiffer joints.

On the other hand, if as you age, your food instead contains 80-90% intact, unprocessed fruits, vegetables, nuts, and seeds, your stomach and intestines would continue to use all available resources, employing good bacteria to produce a variety of acids and ferment, extracting only what our body and bacteria hosts require from the fiber dense intact cells you feed on as sustenance and nutrition. A whole food diet will bring homeostasis to your entire digestive system, right down to your colon and even rectum, or return what is referred to as homeostatic control. [82]

On the other hand, indulgence in a Western diet as you age will slowly place a thin coat of gunk over tissue cells and prevent highly processed sugars, like table sugar, flour, and syrups from being absorbed and used by cells, leaving a kind of crust that repels insulin and oxygen. Combined with a variety of pathogens from meats, toxins from synthetic chemicals and metals, these insults wreak havoc on digestion and circulation and start to damage the organs responsible for metabolism.

Aging on a western diet has many consequences. Slowly, neuropathy starts, from skin itching, acne, and rashes to numbness and pain.[83] Unbeknownst to you, your muscles will start to get squishy, and your bones will hollow out.[84] Eventually, walking starts to become difficult,[85] fluids in the ear calcify,[86] cells responsible for your eyesight become rigid and fail,[87] and lung function decreases.[88] An uneventful common fall caused by clumsiness now fractures bones. Minor cuts or injuries stop healing and turn into amputated limbs.[89] Diseases such as COPD (Chronic Obstructive Pulmonary Disease), and IBS (irritable bowel syndrome) start popping up. Very tiny calcified dead spots, polyps, or lesions start to develop on your skin, throughout your body, and eventually in your brain. Your immune system starts attacking the body and you become a ripe environment for cellular mutinies inside us we call cancer.[90]

These tiny lesions and dead spots are near impossible to heal, very difficult to dissolve, and they start to calcify and block neuronal pathways, leading to degeneration and diseases like Alzheimer's, Parkinson's, and even Multiple Sclerosis.[91] Scientists use terms like *inflamm-aging* or *garb-aging* to describe this progression of metabolic dysfunction.[92] If your Western lifestyle is exceptionally indulgent into your sixties and seventies, you will have blood vessel leaks, plaque buildup, blockages, ruptures, and clots.[93] Some are not so fortunate and have a stroke, but for the rest of us, deterioration is paced.

GENETIC VARIATION

Some people certainly have genetic predispositions that can help to either accelerate or slow down onset. Some of us can eat, drink, and smoke more of the "bad" stuff than others before there is damage or injury. We are all randomly different and the differences between us are why one sibling may be taller, leaner, chubbier, or even smarter. Your spouse or colleague may have slightly better versions of certain genes than you do. He or she may have a less dirty or toxic diet over a lifetime, so there is not as much damage to metabolism.[94] When I was in law school, my best friend was tall and skinny, and if he did not eat three meals a day he would pass out. At the same time, I was short and chubby, and I could go a full twenty-four hours in between a large meal and remain completely satiated. These physical and slight genetic differences are somewhat important in accelerating or preventing the onset of diabetes but don't be discouraged, they are not controlling factors. Diet, toxins, and a sedentary lifestyle are far greater predictors of metabolic dysfunction.

THE SOLUTION

The good news is that a good diet and lifestyle can halt any further deterioration and even slowly reverse any existing damage. You can clean and clear the swampy, pond-like diabetic environment inside you with diet and lifestyle modification, and with some metabolic tweaks, even reverse some cellular level dysfunction over time.[95] There is no other way. There is no magic pill, device, or medical procedure that can fix metabolic dysfunction. Once you change your diet and lifestyle, your metabolism will drastically improve and clear the circulatory paths, get rid of the overpopulation of existing retired cells,[96] and start to reverse the inflammation inside.[97]

---

[52] National Research Council (US) Committee on Diet, Nutrition, and Cancer. Diet, Nutrition, and Cancer: Directions for Research. Washington (DC): National Academies Press (US); 1983. 8, Food Additives, Contaminants, Carcinogens, and Mutagens.

[53] Schulte EM, Avena NM, Gearhardt AN. Which foods may be addictive? The roles of processing, fat content, and glycemic load. *PLoS One*. 2015;10(2):e0117959. Published 2015 Feb 18. doi:10.1371/journal.pone.0117959

[54]George AM, Jacob AG, Fogelfeld L. Lean diabetes mellitus: An emerging entity in the era of obesity. *World J Diabetes*. 2015;6(4):613–620. doi:10.4239/wjd.v6.i4.613

[55] U.S. Department of Health and Human Services. The Health Consequences of Smoking—50 Years of Progress. A Report of the Surgeon General. Atlanta: U.S. DHHS, CDC, NCCDPHP, OSH, 2014.

[56] Smith HS. Opioid metabolism. *Mayo Clin Proc*. 2009;84(7):613-624. doi:10.1016/S0025-6196(11)60750-7

[57] Beaulieu P. Toxic effects of cannabis and cannabinoids: Animal data. *Pain Res Manag*. 2005;10 Suppl A:23A-6A. doi:10.1155/2005/763623

[58] Sullivan EV, Zahr NM. Neuroinflammation as a neurotoxic mechanism in alcoholism: commentary on "Increased MCP-1 and microglia in various regions of human alcoholic brain". *Exp Neurol*. 2008;213(1):10-17. doi:10.1016/j.expneurol.2008.05.016

[59] Nicotine Keeps Leaf-Loving Herbivores at Bay. *PLoS Biol.* 2004;2(8):e250. doi:10.1371/journal.pbio.0020250

[60] Willson C. The clinical toxicology of caffeine: A review and case study. *Toxicol Rep.* 2018;5:1140-1152. Published 2018 Nov 3. doi:10.1016/j.toxrep.2018.11.002

[61] Centers for Disease Control and Prevention. Current Cigarette Smoking Among Adults—United States, 2017. Morbidity and Mortality Weekly Report 2018;67(44):1225-32.

[62] Substance Abuse and Mental Health Services Administration (SAMHSA). 2015 National Survey on Drug Use and Health (NSDUH). Table 2.46B—Alcohol Use, Binge Alcohol Use, and Heavy Alcohol Use in Past Month among Persons Aged 12 or Older, by Demographic Characteristics: Percentages, 2014 and 2015.

[63] Liauchonak I, Qorri B, Dawoud F, Riat Y, Szewczuk MR. Non-Nutritive Sweeteners and Their Implications on the Development of Metabolic Syndrome. *Nutrients.* 2019;11(3):644. Published 2019 Mar 16. doi:10.3390/nu11030644

[64]Pizzorno J. Is the Diabetes Epidemic Primarily Due to Toxins? *Integrative Medicine: A Clinician's Journal.* 2016;15(4):8-17.

[65] Hamilton D, et al.; Advisory Committee on Crop Protection CDCE of the IU PAC. Pesticide residues in food--acute dietary exposure. Pest Manag Sci. 2004 Apr;60(4):311-39. Review.

[66] Samsel A, Seneff S. Glyphosate, pathways to modern diseases II: Celiac sprue and gluten intolerance. *Interdiscip Toxicol.* 2013;6(4):159–184. doi:10.2478/intox-2013-0026

[67] Zahm SH, Blair A. Pesticides and non-Hodgkin's lymphoma. Cancer Res. 1992 Oct 1;52(19 Suppl):5485s-5488s. Review.

[68]Burkholder J, Libra B, Weyer P, et al. Impacts of waste from concentrated animal feeding operations on water quality. *Environ Health Perspect.* 2007;115(2):308–312. doi:10.1289/ehp.8839

[69]Mercola J, Mermer C. Many people are taking insulin-like growth factor-I without even knowing it. *West J Med.* 2001;175(6):378–379.

doi:10.1136/ewjm.175.6.378

[70]Calvo MS, Moshfegh AJ, Tucker KL. Assessing the health impact of phosphorus in the food supply: issues and considerations. *Adv Nutr.* 2014;5(1):104–113. Published 2014 Jan 1. doi:10.3945/an.113.004861

[71]Weber R, et al. Reviewing the relevance of dioxin and PCB sources for food from animal origin and the need for their inventory, control and management. *Environ Sci Eur.* 2018;30(1):42. doi:10.1186/s12302-018-0166-9

[72]Gonçalves-Tenório A, et al. Prevalence of Pathogens in Poultry Meat: A Meta-Analysis of European Published Surveys. *Foods.* 2018;7(5):69. doi:10.3390/foods7050069.

[73]Marshall BM, Levy SB. Food Animals and Antimicrobials: Impacts on Human Health. *Clinical Microbiology Reviews.* 2011;24(4):718-733. doi:10.1128/CMR.00002-11.\\

[74]Lahou E, et al.. Effectiveness of inactivation of foodborne pathogensInt J Food Microbiol. 2015 Aug 3;206:118-29. doi: 10.1016/j.ijfoodmicro.2015.04.014. Epub 2015 Apr 11. PMID: 26004267

[75]Yan D, Zhang Y, Liu L, Yan H. Pesticide exposure and risk of Alzheimer's disease: a systematic review and meta-analysis. *Sci Rep.* 2016;6:32222. Published 2016 Sep 1. doi:10.1038/srep32222

[76]Ahmed H, Abushouk AI, Gabr M, Negida A, Abdel-Daim MM. Parkinson's disease and pesticides BiomedPharmacother. 2017 Jun;90:638-649. doi: 10.1016/j.biopha.2017.03.100. Epub 2017 Apr 14.

[77] Kandimalla R, Thirumala V, Reddy PH. Is Alzheimer's disease a Type 3 Diabetes? A critical appraisal. *BiochimBiophysActaMol Basis Dis.* 2017;1863(5):1078–1089. doi:10.1016/j.bbadis.2016.08.018

[78] Danielson ML, Bitsko RH, Ghandour RM, Holbrook JR, Kogan MD, Blumberg SJ. Prevalence of Parent-Reported ADHD Diagnosis and Associated Treatment Among U.S. Children and Adolescents, 2016. *J Clin Child Adolesc Psychol.* 2018;47(2):199–212. doi:10.1080/15374416.2017.1417860

[79] Fuhrman J. The Hidden Dangers of Fast and Processed Food. *Am J Lifestyle Med.* 2018;12(5):375–381. Published 2018 Apr 3. doi:10.1177/1559827618766483

[80]Gearhardt AN, Grilo CM, DiLeone RJ, Brownell KD, Potenza MN.Can Food

be Addictive? Public Health and Policy Implications. *Addiction (Abingdon, England)*. 2011;106(7):1208-1212. doi:10.1111/j.1360-0443.2010.03301.x.

[81]DeBerardinis RJ, Thompson CB. Cellular metabolism and disease: what do metabolic outliers teach us?. *Cell.* 2012;148(6):1132–1144. doi:10.1016/j.cell.2012.02.032

[82]Glick-Bauer M, Yeh M-C. The Health Advantage of a Vegan Diet: Exploring the Gut Microbiota Connection. *Nutrients.* 2014;6(11):4822-4838. doi:10.3390/nu6114822.

[83] Rajchgot T, Thomas SC, Wang JC, et al. Neurons and Microglia; A Sickly-Sweet Duo in Diabetic Pain Neuropathy. *Front Neurosci.* 2019;13:25. Published 2019 Jan 31. doi:10.3389/fnins.2019.00025

[84] Greco EA, Pietschmann P, Migliaccio S. Osteoporosis and Sarcopenia Increase Frailty Syndrome in the Elderly. *Front Endocrinol (Lausanne).* 2019;10:255. Published 2019 Apr 24. doi:10.3389/fendo.2019.00255

[85] Abate M, Schiavone C, Salini V, Andia I. Management of limited joint mobility in diabetic patients. *Diabetes Metab Syndr Obes.* 2013;6:197–207. Published 2013 May 7. doi:10.2147/DMSO.S33943

[86] Bainbridge KE, Hoffman HJ, Cowie CC. Diabetes and hearing impairment in the United States: audiometric evidence from the National Health and Nutrition Examination Survey, 1999 to 2004. *Ann Intern Med.* 2008;149(1):1–10. doi:10.7326/0003-4819-149-1-200807010-00231

[87]Diabetic retinopathy preferred practice pattern guidelines. American Academy of Ophthalmology website. https://www.aao.org/preferred-practice-pattern/diabetic-retinopathy-ppp-updated-2016.

[88] Pitocco D, Fuso L, Conte EG, et al. The diabetic lung--a new target organ?. *Rev Diabet Stud.* 2012;9(1):23–35. doi:10.1900/RDS.2012.9.23

[89] Huang YY, et al. Survival and associated risk factors in patients with diabetes and amputations caused by infectious foot gangrene. *J Foot Ankle Res.* 2018;11:1. Published 2018 Jan 4. doi:10.1186/s13047-017-0243-0.

[90] Kubben N, Misteli T. Shared molecular and cellular mechanisms of premature ageing and ageing-associated diseases. *Nat Rev Mol Cell Biol.*

2017;18(10):595–609. doi:10.1038/nrm.2017.68

[91] Castillo X, Castro-Obregón S, Gutiérrez-Becker B, et al. Re-thinking the Etiological Framework of Neurodegeneration. *Front Neurosci.* 2019;13:728. Published 2019 Jul 24. doi:10.3389/fnins.2019.00728

[92] Franceschi C, Garagnani P, Vitale G, Capri M, Salvioli S. Inflammaging and 'Garb-aging'. Trends Endocrinol Metab. 2017 Mar;28 (3):199-212. doi: 10.1016/j.tem.2016.09.005. Epub 2016 Oct 24. Review.

[93]Hajjar DP, Gotto AM. Biological Relevance of Inflammation and Oxidative Stress in the Pathogenesis of Arterial Diseases. *The American Journal of Pathology.* 2013;182(5):1474-1481. doi:10.1016/j.ajpath.2013.01.010.

[94] Zhang W, Xin L, Lu Y. Integrative Analysis to Identify Common Genetic Markers of Metabolic Syndrome, Dementia, and Diabetes. *Med Sci Monit.* 2017;23:5885–5891. Published 2017 Dec 12. doi:10.12659/msm.905521

[95]Burton DGA, Faragher RGA. Obesity and type-2 diabetes as inducers of premature cellular senescence and ageing. *Biogerontology.* 2018;19(6):447–459. doi:10.1007/s10522-018-9763-7

[96]Freund A, Orjalo AV, Desprez P-Y, Campisi J. Inflammatory Networks during Cellular Senescence: Causes and Consequences. *Trends in molecular medicine.* 2010;16(5):238-246.

[97]Hobson S, Arefin S, Kublickiene K, Shiels PG, Stenvinkel P. Senescent Cells in Early Vascular Ageing and Bone Disease of Chronic Kidney Disease-A Novel Target for Treatment. *Toxins (Basel).* 2019;11(2):82. Published 2019 Feb 1. doi:10.3390/toxins11020082.

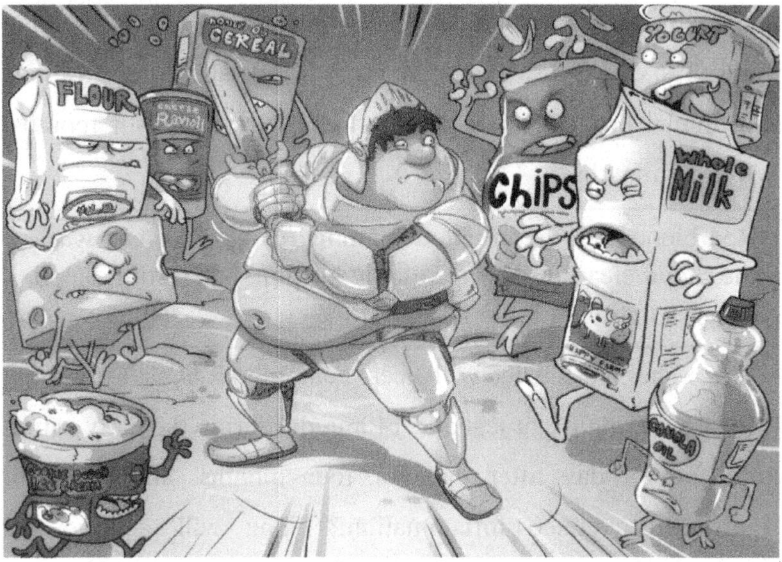

CHAPTER 3

THE WASH CYCLE DIET

In 1982, Ms. Ann Wigmore published a recipe book called *Recipes for Longer Life*. She predicted the diabetes health crisis we are in now. She wrote "modern living, with its cooked food, overstimulation, and destructive living habits has made of our bodies clogged sewage systems."[98] There are probably thousands of scientific studies and articles written since then that have validated her claim. Her book gave me the inspiration for the Wash Cycle Diet (WC Diet) created here.

The Wash Cycle Diet is designed to keep you full but not drowsily satiated, free of synthetic chemicals, and free of foods that compromise metabolism (complex proteins, cholesterol, and oxidation products). The Wash Cycle diet avoids hunger by filling up with digestion-neutral or calorie-negative foods. The diet is a raw plant diet that avoids all processed foods and animal products. We do this for a period of four months. Why four months?

> Red blood cells live for four months (cycle). We can wash the blood clean during a cycle by keeping our fasting blood sugar at optimal levels.

The Wash Diet will keep your blood sugar at optimal levels (85-95mg/dL at fast and 140mg/dL during the daily eating time frame), day after day for four months, and this will significantly reduce inflammation.[99] You will deprive the bloodstream of ultra-processed easily absorbed sugars like flour, milk, syrup, and table sugar.

Years of waxy oily foods have built up foamy coats of fat all throughout your body. This fat blocks insulin from unlocking your cells. Insulin resistance causes erratic and unmanageable spikes in blood sugar levels. So just avoiding easily dissolvable sugars like table sugar, syrup, flour, and milk is not enough. The Wash Cycle diet will reduce your constant triglyceride/cholesterol blood levels by eliminating animal products and all oils from your diet.

> Constantly high cholesterol and triglyceride levels bring about insulin resistance. No more meat and fried or oily

To further help dissolve the crystals, remnants, proteins, foam, and oxides (gunk), and to use up existing subcutaneous fats that promote diabetes, the Wash Diet forces the body into autophagy through fasting for a few hours every day. The diet uses raw food to restrict calories and employs light intermittent fasting, giving the body time between feedings to dissolve and burn gunk.

Eat one large raw meal a day which will restrict calories and fast in between meals to promote autophagy.

Finally, to prevent future metabolic deterioration, we must stop damage to metabolic organs. The Wash Cycle Diet is designed to stop the onslaught of daily toxins we are exposed to. You will eliminate pesticides, fryer oil, heavily grilled charring, and pathogens from the diet. You will also stop or significantly reduce intake of drugs that have negative effects on metabolism like caffeine,[100] alcohol,[101] THC,[102] and nicotine.[103]

Stop toxins and pathogens from getting into your body to stop further damage to organs responsible for metabolism.

CHOLESTEROL, OIL, ANIMAL FAT, AND ANIMAL PROTEIN

The first major important diet correction will require the elimination of animal products and oil from your diet. Fat makes food delicious but also provides very easy calories that are hard to dispose of. One cup of oil has 2,000 easily absorbed and readily storable calories.[104] Fats are most dangerous when they accumulate in the liver[105] and in pockets in tissue.[106] Imagine a sort of marbling effect in your muscles.[107] Depending on the type of fat, and where the fat is in your body, fat blocks circulation and fat cells excrete hormones that promote diabetes mellitus.[108]

Examples of processed fats that are toxic and dangerous are lard, fryer oil, butter, melted coconut oil, and even the most organic cold-pressed, antioxidant-packed olive oil. Animal products are also a major source of cholesterol. As you age, assume that all animal fats and processed oils are bad for you and treat them as a once-in-a-while delicacy that you ingest in very small portions.[109] Studies have shown detectible increases in blood pressure from arterial stiffening for a four-hour period after a meal high in fat.[110] Stiffening of blood pathways happens even after consumption of very supposedly light oils filled with antioxidants,[111] like olive or avocado oil.[112] Even vegetarian diets where a sizable portion of the diet comes from oils and frying to add flavor are very dangerous to the health of an aging pre-diabetic or diabetic.[113] The Wash Cycle Diet is designed to eliminate high cholesterol animal products (meat, cheese, eggs) and fryer oil prepared foods (chips, nuggets, onion rings, French fries),[114] as well as oil-based products such as mayonnaise, oil-infused dressings, and sauces.

When I talk about this lifestyle change to folks, the first question they always ask is "*What do you do for protein?*"[115] This is the wrong question to ask. The better question is "*What type of protein are you consuming*?" Studies show that diets high in animal proteins accelerate the onset of diabetes mellitus.[116] There is also a mistaken belief that high protein diets are essential for older people.[117] People also erroneously believe that animal-based proteins are a more complete source of protein.[118] There is no question that meats and eggs contain high levels of complex branched chain amino acids[119] and high levels of cholesterol.[120] When these animal products like milk, cheese, eggs, and meat are aged, heated, cooled, and reheated, or when you fry in oil, unhealthy oxides develop.[121]

If you ever strictly followed a Keto, Atkins, or South Beach-style diet, you probably have noticed some immediate adverse effects that should raise alarms: dehydration, electrolyte imbalance, headaches, digestive tract rotting, bad breath, unpleasant gas, leg cramps, and diarrhea.

Although people claim that these diets help them lose weight, studies have not shown that a diet high in animal fat/protein and low in carbohydrates actually brings about sustained weight loss.[122] There is certainly no question that these diets lower A1c levels because they starve the body of sugar carbohydrates.[123] But a pre-diabetic or diabetic is more concerned with blood triglyceride, cholesterol levels, and oxidation products in the long term because fats and oxides block insulin receptors. High animal fat/protein diets actually increase blood cholesterol levels,[124] which in turn increase insulin resistance.[125] As muscle is processed, cooked, fried, caramelized, dehydrated, and re-heated, the end result is an oxidized food product that, according to the World Health Organization, is as unhealthy for you as smoking cigarettes.[126] A variety of animal and human studies have shown that red or processed meats are an independent cause of metabolic disorder,[127] contribute to certain digestive tract cancers,[128] and are major contributors to vascular disease.[129]

As we age, we also naturally lose kidney function[130] and the kidneys have a hard time disposing of complex proteins.[131] Too much protein can also hollow out bones,[132] and clog arteries.[133] We know that mice fed a low protein, high carbohydrate diet live longer.[134] So the Wash Cycle Diet is designed to eliminate the smorgasbord of easily digestible calories that come from animal products and oils,[135] and replace oxidized products with raw unrefined plant fats and proteins. Fat and protein found naturally in plants provide an abundance of raw unfiltered plant-based omega fatty acids and essential amino acids.[136]

During the Wash Cycle Diet, and hopefully, for the rest of your life, you will source fats from raw nuts,[137] such as walnuts,[138] or other plants like avocados,[139] coconuts,[140] olives,[141] chia, and flax seeds.[142] These natural unprocessed omega fats will help reverse plaque formation, oxidative stress, and inflammation.[143] You can also indulge occasionally and consume raw plant milks and nut butters. But remember that even plant milk and butter are somewhat processed. There are also plenty of protein in plants sources,[144] and the wash cycle diet sources protein from cooked legumes (beans),[145] which also naturally help (producing gas) to keep your digestive tract clean and healthy.[146]

CARBOHYDRATES

Our main source of energy, as humans, is carbohydrates, but what you really need as you get older is raw plant fiber.[147] Our goal, as we age, is to reduce digestibility and increase raw fiber consumption.[148] The Wash Cycle Diet eliminates ultra-processed carbohydrates[149] and replaces them with raw, plant-based, and uncooked carbohydrates that will not melt in your mouth and absorb easily.[150]

Processed foods are deceptively high in simple sugars. A glass of milk has about as much sugar as a candy bar. One half of a cup of store-bought spaghetti sauce has as much sugar as a donut. An eight-ounce cup of fruit juice has twice the sugar of a candy bar. Liquid calories are especially bad for you because a very small amount can pack a very big punch. Calorie-packed liquids are supercharged and easily absorb into the bloodstream. On the other hand, a banana, grape, or date is far less digestible. Although fruits are full of sugar, raw fruit has a neutral effect on digestion and weight gain because most of the sugar in fruit is still unprocessed.[151] Only when you process fruit and extract its sugars by juicing do you make those sugars easily accessible.[152]

Imagine carbohydrates as being either bushes or trees. The bush has many thin and weak branches, while the tree has thick and strong branches. An easily digestible carbohydrate (a "bush") would be high fructose corn syrup, table sugar, milk, fruit juice, and flour. Look at pizza dough, chocolate, cake, or any other foods that are processed and then cooked. Your body will easily digest the super processed weak branches in these foods causing a massive flood of simple sugars to enter the bloodstream.

On the other hand, uncooked fruits and vegetables, or raw nuts and seeds are hard to digest and rich in fiber (the "trees"). These raw fibers have fewer and thicker branches, thereby requiring far more effort to break down. You might think that mashed potatoes or cooked vegetables are healthier than eating pizza or a hamburger,[153] and you are not wrong, because we are eliminating the most digestible flours, sugars, oils, and cholesterol, but the goal of the Wash Cycle Diet is to clean and clear, therefore we also need to eliminate as many easy to digest cooked or processed carbohydrates as we can for the four-month duration of the diet.

> The Wash Cycle Diet will also eliminate all sources of highly digestible carbohydrates. The goal is to keep your carbohydrates as intact and full of raw fiber as possible.

With raw plant-based carbohydrates, very little of the simple sugars actually get absorbed into the bloodstream and most of what you eat will move down the digestive tract where a healthy microbiome will convert the raw fibers into exotic molecules that will nurture optimum metabolism.[154] Over ninety percent of your new diet will now be raw, hard-to-digest plants, creating a natural form of caloric restriction, allowing your body to start cleaning and clearing without hunger, starvation, or nutritional deficiency. This reduced digestibility is the cornerstone of the Wash Cycle Diet,[155] and it acts to restrict calories, which when combined with a reduced daily window of consumption (intermittent fasting discussed later in the chapter), will allow metabolic autophagy or self-devouring. By restricting caloric intake by 25% for 24 months, there can be a persistent reduction in inflammatory markers by as much as 50%.[156]

SATIETY

There is no question that the first few weeks on a raw plant diet will be challenging. You will feel hungry more often and less satisfied, sometimes even after you eat a pound of raw carbohydrates. Raw food lacks the pleasure punch that processed and cooked fats and proteins provide. This is exactly why processed foods are addictive because the good feeling you get is comparable to using drugs, alcohol, tobacco, or caffeine. For 40 or more years, you have been chasing that daily food high and it will take a good amount of willpower before that less than full feeling goes unnoticed. But you will never go hungry on the Wash Cycle Diet, and over a period of just a couple of weeks, you will stop missing that comatose feeling you got after a Western meal.

> Even after the Wash Cycle Diet, and for the rest of your life, your diet should be 75% raw fruits, vegetables and nuts.

TOXINS AND ORGANIC VEGETABLES AND FRUITS

Folks who eat organic have a lower incidence of diabetes.[157] Chronic exposure to fryer oil, cooking, pesticides, synthetic perfumes, hormones, or other unnatural products like plastics, metals, and pollution can seriously damage your vital organs. I recently read that we each eat as much as a credit card's worth of micro-plastics a week.[158]

So what is organic? According to the National Organic Standards Board, organic means that "materials and practices" were used "that enhance the ecological balance of natural systems and that integrate the parts of the farming system into an ecological whole."[159] The USDA seal means your produce was certified to be free of synthetic pesticides/fertilizers, genetically engineered ingredients, antibiotics, artificial hormones, and the use of sewage sludge as irrigation. The farmland must be clear of prohibited substances for at least three years, crops must be rotated regularly, and seeds must be organically grown. Regulations mandate that only a couple of dozen mostly natural pesticides, herbicides, and fungicides can be used to grow organic produce.[160] Organic diet intervention can reduce body pesticide excretion by as much as 95% in as little as six days.[161]

If food cost is an important factor for you, keep in mind that some fruits and vegetables are not treated with chemicals and pesticides, such as onions, broccoli, mushrooms, asparagus, cabbage, and cantaloupes. Many fruits can also be peeled. Finally, you can neutralize virtually all the pesticides that are sprayed on most fruits and vegetables by soaking them in a mixture of water and baking soda (sodium bicarbonate) for a few minutes.[162] Baking soda is a great alkalizing agent.

By eliminating cooking, toxic fryer oils, and plastic fibers, you will make a positive difference, and along with switching to an organic diet, you will eliminate the intake of all synthetic chemicals and stop any further damage to delicate aging organs responsible for metabolism.

INTERMITTENT FASTING

Starving is very effective at ending diabetes because it's a "complete" approach, but it is obviously not a permanent or safely sustainable solution. One of the major goals of the Wash Cycle Diet is to give the body time between feedings to self-devour without starvation. This is achieved by eating a lot of food (maybe up to two to four pounds of raw carbohydrates) in a short period of time (let's say between 12:00 pm and 5:00 pm) and then fasting until the next day. Raw food is digestion-neutral/negative-creating natural caloric restriction, and along with *intermittent* fasting for 18 to 22 hours in between feedings, we force the body to self-devour (autophagy).[163]

Intermittent fasting will allow enough time between feedings to clean and clear your body.[164] Animal studies have shown that mice fed one meal a day live longer,[165] and intermittent fasting has been shown to reverse diabetes in animals.[166] Such a modest dietary adjustment, limiting eating to one meal a day or even to between four or even six hours during the day, can make a significant difference in your health.[167] Scientists now regularly suggest that we fast intermittently.[168]

The Wash Cycle Diet tries to find the right balance. To get the full effect of intermittent fasting, you need to fast for two to three days, but this is not reasonable for older diabetics. By limiting food consumption to one large continuous meal a day that stretches for four hours,[169] and feeding on foods that naturally create caloric restriction, you will achieve modest cleaning and clearing.[170] Start with an eight hour per day window of eating and set a goal to get down to a four hour per day window of eating within a couple weeks.

BECOMING A CENTENARIAN

The diet of most successful centenarians promotes autophagy, keeps a clean cellular environment, contains sufficient micronutrients,[171] and avoids toxins. A raw, fiber-rich plant diet will provide natural calorie restriction while improving health,[172] intermittent fasting will allow the body time to clean and clear,[173] and a few tweaks we'll discuss later will improve the function of metabolism.[174] Your body will reward you by removing much of the excess accumulated waste stored up in the body.[175]

We all have different metabolism rates and we still have much to learn about metabolism and aging,[176] but what matters here is that you understand that it will be difficult for some of you with faster metabolism to sustain a lifetime 90% raw plant diet coupled with an 18 to 22 hour fast between feedings.[177]

After the Wash Cycle Diet, if you just can't do it, then experiment with different diet consistencies and fasting intervals. If you start feeling hunger too fast, increase your window of consumption, or the amount of cooked vegetables you consume until you find the right balance that gets you through until the next day's eating cycle. Sometimes, when my body gives me that strong desire for something denser and fattier, I will make a bean and rice plate. The purpose of a raw plant diet is to get you healthy, not to torture, so if you need a little extra boost of carbohydrates because you crave it, satisfy the urge in moderation. The Wash Cycle is about cleaning and clearing, and if you remain strict for a long time, your body will let you know. You will walk by a bakery and be drawn to the smell. For those with a fast metabolism or that work on their feet and with their hands all day, if most of your diet is raw fruits, vegetables, nuts, and seeds that are free of processing, oil, cholesterol, and complex proteins, you can still eat some cooked grains and vegetables to keep hunger at bay. The goal here is to achieve calorie restriction, clean eating, and autophagy safely for four months, not for you to pass out or feel hungry all day.

A strict four-month Wash Cycle will reduce most people's body weight by as much as 20%, and for some, this weight loss may be very welcome. But for older diabetics of average weight and Body Mass Index (BMI), your goal is not weight loss, and instead, your focus should be on *clean* eating. In your case, you may not be able to sustain four straight months of a wash cycle, so you either must add additional doses of *clean* energy (some lightly cooked vegetables, cooked whole rice, grains, or legumes, or semi-processed carbohydrates like nut butter) in order to achieve fullness, or you will need to increase the daily feeding window timeframe. Start by increasing the number of cooked legumes you eat. If that doesn't do it, add raw nut butter and plant milk to your diet. If that doesn't do it, increase the percentage of steamed or boiled vegetables or whole grains, like quinoa.[178] You can also include a tablespoon or two of raw cold-pressed olive or avocado oil in your dressings. Quantity is less important when you eat raw. You can eat from two to four pounds of raw plants during a daily feeding window and still clean and clear. You can adjust the diet to find the right balance, where the feeling of hunger goes away long enough to make it to the next day. Just remember, that addictive feeling of satiety that comes from processed foods and animal products will be hard to shake off and like most addicts, it will take a couple of weeks before your body stops craving those ultra-rich foods.

Now, as a last note, let's be clear that this fasting does not apply to water consumption. Later we talk about how important water consumption is, and you should drink about half of your weight in water ounces every day. To spice it up, you can drink most green teas, naturally decaffeinated coffees, fruit-flavored bubbly waters, or any other water that has not been sweetened with any synthetic chemicals. You can sweeten your drink with a couple of dates, raisins, or figs.

The Wash Cycle Diet duration is four months or until all the test results from chapter one come back to normal, whichever is longer. Once everything is normal and you are satisfied with how much you weigh, you can create more of a hybrid diet where you increase cooked rice and whole grains, steamed vegetables, or maybe even add some oven-roasted fish or boiled eggs, but keep a continuous eye on your vitals. For the rest of your life meats, frying, oils, sugar, cheese, animal milk, eggs, and flour (even coconut or nut flours) are to be considered delicacies for an *occasional* indulgence.

---

[98]Wigmore, A. Recipes for Longer Life, Avery (1982).

[99] Temelkova-Kurktschiev T, Siegert G, Bergmann S, et al. Subclinical inflammation is strongly related to insulin resistance but not to impaired insulin secretion in a high risk population for diabetes. *Metabolism.* 2002;51(6):743-749. doi:10.1053/meta.2002.32804

[100] Willson C. The clinical toxicology of caffeine: A review and case study. *Toxicol Rep.* 2018;5:1140-1152. Published 2018 Nov 3. doi:10.1016/j.toxrep.2018.11.002

[101] Leonard BE. Is ethanol a neurotoxin?: The effects of ethanol on neuronal structure and function. *Alcohol Alcohol.* 1986;21(4):325-338.

[102] Kelly BF, Nappe TM. Cannabinoid Toxicity. [Updated 2019 Sep 6]. In: StatPearls [Internet]. Treasure Island (FL): StatPearls Publishing; 2020 Jan-. Available from: https://www.ncbi.nlm.nih.gov/books/NBK482175/

[103] Mishra A, Chaturvedi P, Datta S, Sinukumar S, Joshi P, Garg A. Harmful effects of nicotine. *Indian J Med Paediatr Oncol.* 2015;36(1):24-31.

doi:10.4103/0971-5851.151771

[104] Groopman EE, Carmody RN, Wrangham RW. Cooking increases net energy gain from a lipid-rich food. *Am J Phys Anthropol.* 2015;156(1):11–18. doi:10.1002/ajpa.22622

[105] Püschel GP, Henkel J. Dietary cholesterol does not break your heart but kills your liver. *Porto Biomed J.* 2019;3(1):e12. Published 2019 Jun 29. doi:10.1016/j.pbj.0000000000000012

[106] Chait A, den Hartigh LJ. Adipose Tissue Distribution, Inflammation and Its Metabolic Consequences, Including Diabetes and Cardiovascular Disease. *Front Cardiovasc Med.* 2020;7:22. Published 2020 Feb 25. doi:10.3389/fcvm.2020.00022

[107] Chait A, den Hartigh LJ. Adipose Tissue Distribution, Inflammation and Its Metabolic Consequences, Including Diabetes and Cardiovascular Disease. *Front Cardiovasc Med.* 2020;7:22. Published 2020 Feb 25. doi:10.3389/fcvm.2020.00022

[108] Madhusoodanan J. The Secret Life of Fat Cells. *ACS Cent Sci.* 2018;4(9):1078–1080. doi:10.1021/acscentsci.8b00633

[109] Khan MI, Min JS, Lee SO, et al. Cooking, storage, and reheating effect on the formation of cholesterol oxidation products in processed meat products. *Lipids Health Dis.* 2015;14:89. Published 2015 Aug 11. doi:10.1186/s12944-015-0091-5

[110] Lithander FE, Herlihy LK, Walsh DM, Burke E, Crowley V, Mahmud A. Postprandial effect of dietary fat quantity and quality on arterial stiffness and wave reflection: a randomised controlled trial. *Nutr J.* 2013;12:93. Published 2013 Jul 10. doi:10.1186/1475-2891-12-93

[111]Hamley S. The effect of replacing saturated fat with mostly n-6 polyunsaturated fat on coronary heart disease: a meta-analysis of randomised controlled trials. *Nutrition Journal.* 2017;16:30. doi:10.1186/s12937-017-0254-

[112] Vogel RA. Brachial artery ultrasound: a noninvasive tool in the assessment of triglyceride-rich lipoproteins. *Clin Cardiol.* 1999;22(6 Suppl):II34–II39. doi:10.1002/clc.4960221407

[113] Olfert MD, Wattick RA. Vegetarian Diets and the Risk of Diabetes. *Curr*

Diab Rep. 2018;18(11):101. Published 2018 Sep 18. doi:10.1007/s11892-018-1070-9

[114] PerumallaVenkata R, Subramanyam R. Evaluation of the deleterious health effects of consumption of repeatedly heated vegetable oil. *Toxicology Reports*. 2016;3:636-643.

[115] Mariotti F, Gardner CD. Dietary Protein and Amino Acids in Vegetarian Diets-A Review. *Nutrients*. 2019;11(11):2661. Published 2019 Nov 4. doi:10.3390/nu11112661

[116] Zhao LG, Zhang QL, Liu XL, Wu H, Zheng JL, Xiang YB. Dietary protein intake and risk of type 2 diabetes: a dose-response meta-analysis of prospective studies. *Eur J Nutr*. 2019;58(4):1351-1367. doi:10.1007/s00394-018-1737-7

[117] Verreijen AM, Engberink MF, Houston DK, et al. Dietary protein intake is not associated with 5-y change in mid-thigh muscle cross-sectional area by computed tomography in older adults: the Health, Aging, and Body Composition (Health ABC) Study. *Am J Clin Nutr*. 2019;109(3):535-543. doi:10.1093/ajcn/nqy341

[118] Mariotti F. Plant protein, animal protein, and protein quality. Vegetarian and Plant-Based Diets in Health and Disease Prevention. Academic Press; Cambridge, MA, USA: 2017. pp. 621–642.

[119] Fan M, Li Y, Wang C, et al. Dietary Protein Consumption and the Risk of Type 2 Diabetes: ADose-Response Meta-Analysis of Prospective Studies. *Nutrients*. 2019;11(11):2783. Published 2019 Nov 15. doi:10.3390/nu11112783

[120] O'Neill B, Raggi P. The ketogenic diet: Pros and cons. *Atherosclerosis*. 2020;292:119-126. doi:10.1016/j.atherosclerosis.2019.11.021

[121] Otaegui-Arrazola A, Menéndez-Carreño M, Ansorena D, Astiasarán I.Oxysterols: A world to explore. Food Chem Toxicol. 2010 Dec;48(12):3289-303. doi: 10.1016/j.fct.2010.09.023. Epub 2010 Sep 24. Review.

[122] Seid H, Rosenbaum M. Low Carbohydrate and Low-Fat Diets: What We Don't Know and Why we Should Know It. *Nutrients*. 2019;11(11):2749. Published 2019 Nov 12. doi:10.3390/nu11112749

[123] Clemente Fuentes RW, Broszko CM, Pietralcyzk ES, Nashelsky J. Efficacy of a low-carbohydrate or ketogenic diet in preventing patient morbidity and mortality. *Can Fam Physician.* 2020;66(4):262-263.

[124] Kwiterovich PO Jr, Vining EP, Pyzik P, Skolasky R Jr, Freeman JM. Effect of a high-fat ketogenic diet on plasma levels of lipids, lipoproteins, and apolipoproteins in children. *JAMA.* 2003;290(7):912-920. doi:10.1001/jama.290.7.912

[125] Kawamoto R, Tabara Y, Kohara K, et al. Relationships between lipid profiles and metabolic syndrome, insulin resistance and serum high molecular adiponectin in Japanese community-dwelling adults. *Lipids Health Dis.* 2011;10:79. Published 2011 May 17. doi:10.1186/1476-511X-10-79

[126] Zec S, Minto C, Agostoni C, et al. Communicating Risk Regarding Food Consumption: The Case of Processed Meat. *Nutrients.* 2019;11(2):400. Published 2019 Feb 14. doi:10.3390/nu11020400

[127] Tian S, Xu Q, Jiang R, Han T, Sun C, Na L. Dietary Protein Consumption and the Risk of Type 2 Diabetes: A Systematic Review and Meta-Analysis of Cohort Studies. *Nutrients.* 2017;9(9):982. Published 2017 Sep 6. doi:10.3390/nu9090982

[128]Zhang S, Wang Q, He J. Intake of red and processed meat and risk of renal cell carcinoma: a meta-analysis of observational studies. *Oncotarget.* 2017;8(44):77942-77956. doi:10.18632/oncotarget.18549.

[129]David Spence J. Dietary cholesterol and egg yolk should be avoided by patients at risk of vascular disease. *Journal of Translational Internal Medicine.* 2016;4(1):20-24. doi:10.1515/jtim-2016-0005.

[130] Amaral TLM, Amaral CA, Vasconcellos MTL, Monteiro GTR. Prevalence and factors associated to chronic kidney disease in older adults. *Rev Saude Publica.* 2019;53:44. doi:10.11606/S1518-8787.2019053000727

[131] Piccoli GB, Capizzi I, Vigotti FN, et al. Low protein diets in patients with chronic kidney disease: a bridge between mainstream and complementary-alternative medicines?. *BMC Nephrol.* 2016;17(1):76. Published 2016 Jul 8. doi:10.1186/s12882-016-0275-x

[132] Bihuniak JD, Insogna KL. The effects of dietary protein and amino acids on skeletal metabolism. *Mol Cell Endocrinol.* 2015;410:78–86. doi:10.1016/j.mce.2015.03.024

[133] Fleming RM. The effect of high-protein diets on coronary blood flow. Angiology. 2000 Oct;51(10):817-26.

[134]Solon-Biet S. et al. (2014). The ratio of macronutrients, not caloric intake, dictates cardiometabolic health, aging, and longevity in *ad libitum*-fed mice. Cell Metabolism, 19, 418430. https://doi.org/10.1016/j.cmet.2014.02.009

[135] Hall KD, Bemis T, Brychta R, et al. Calorie for Calorie, Dietary Fat Restriction Results in More Body Fat Loss than Carbohydrate Restriction in People with Obesity. *Cell Metab.* 2015;22(3):427-436. doi:10.1016/j.cmet.2015.07.021

[136]Clatici VG, Voicu C, Voaides C, Roseanu A, Icriverzi M, Jurcoane S. Diseases of Civilization - Cancer, Diabetes, Obesity and Acne - the Implication of Milk, IGF-1 and mTORC1. *Maedica (Buchar).* 2018;13(4):273–281. doi:10.26574/maedica.2018.13.4.273

[137] Guasch-Ferré M, Liu X, Malik VS, et al. Nut Consumption and Risk of Cardiovascular Disease. *J Am Coll Cardiol.* 2017;70(20):2519–2532. doi:10.1016/j.jacc.2017.09.035

[138] Katz DL, Davidhi A, Ma Y, Kavak Y, Bifulco L, Njike VY. Effects of walnuts on endothelial function in overweight adults with visceral obesity: a randomized, controlled, crossover trial. *J Am Coll Nutr.* 2012;31(6):415–423. doi:10.1080/07315724.2012.10720468

[139] Park E, Edirisinghe I, Burton-Freeman B. Avocado Fruit on Postprandial Markers of Cardio-Metabolic Risk: A Randomized Controlled Dose Response Trial in Overweight and Obese Men and Women. *Nutrients.* 2018;10(9):1287. Published 2018 Sep 12. doi:10.3390/nu10091287

[140] Ekanayaka RA, Ekanayaka NK, Perera B, De Silva PG. Impact of a traditional dietary supplement with coconut milk and soya milk on the lipid profile in normal free living subjects. *J Nutr Metab.* 2013;2013:481068. doi:10.1155/2013/481068

[141]Ryan, D, Robards, K. Phenolic compounds in olives. Analyst, May 1998,

Vol. 123 (31R–44R). Available at https://pdfs.semanticscholar.org/24b1/54c03d2139150ef66f6e8f1178dde139524a.pdf

142 Kulczyński B, Kobus-Cisowska J, Taczanowski M, Kmiecik D, Gramza-Michałowska A. The Chemical Composition and Nutritional Value of Chia Seeds-Current State of Knowledge. *Nutrients*. 2019;11(6):1242. Published 2019 May 31. doi:10.3390/nu11061242

143 Granic A, Sayer AA, Robinson SM. Dietary Patterns, Skeletal Muscle Health, and Sarcopenia in Older Adults. *Nutrients*. 2019;11(4):745. Published 2019 Mar 30. doi:10.3390/nu11040745

144 Hanjani NA, Vafa M. Protein Restriction, Epigenetic Diet, Intermittent Fasting as New Approaches for Preventing Age-associated Diseases. *Int J Prev Med*. 2018;9:58. Published 2018 Jun 29. doi:10.4103/ijpvm.IJPVM_397_16

145 Margier M, Georgé S, Hafnaoui N, et al. Nutritional Composition and Bioactive Content of Legumes: Characterization of Pulses Frequently Consumed in France and Effect of the Cooking Method. *Nutrients*. 2018;10(11):1668. Published 2018 Nov 4. doi:10.3390/nu10111668

146 Madsen L, Myrmel LS, Fjære E, Liaset B, Kristiansen K. Links between Dietary Protein Sources, the Gut Microbiota, and Obesity. *Front Physiol*. 2017;8:1047. Published 2017 Dec 19. doi:10.3389/fphys.2017.01047

147 Grundy MM-L, Edwards CH, Mackie AR, Gidley MJ, Butterworth PJ, Ellis PR. Re-evaluation of the mechanisms of dietary fibre and implications for macronutrient bioaccessibility, digestion and postprandial metabolism. *The British Journal of Nutrition*. 2016;116(5):816-833. doi:10.1017/S0007114516002610.

148 Higgins JA. Resistant starch and energy balance: impact on weight loss and maintenance. *Critical reviews in food science and nutrition*. 2014;54(9):1158-1166. doi:10.1080/10408398.2011.629352.

149 Hall KD, et al. Ultra-processed diets cause excess calorie intake and weight gain: A one-month inpatient randomized controlled trial of ad libitum food intake. *Cell Metabolism*. May 16, 2019.

150 Kevin D. Hall, KD, Guo, J Pathogenesis of Obesity; Obesity Energetics: Body Weight Regulation and the Effects of Diet Composition. (2017) 152 GASENT 7 1718-1727.e3

[151] Guyenet SJ. Impact of Whole, Fresh Fruit Consumption on Energy Intake and Adiposity: A Systematic Review. *Front Nutr.* 2019;6:66. Published 2019 May 8. doi:10.3389/fnut.2019.00066

[152]Lustig RH. Fructose: It's "Alcohol Without the Buzz." *Advances in Nutrition*. 2013;4(2):226-235. doi:10.3945/an.112.002998.

[153] Chan Q, Stamler J, Brown IJ, et al. Relation of raw and cooked vegetable consumption to blood pressure: the INTERMAP Study. *J Hum Hypertens.* 2014;28(6):353–359. doi:10.1038/jhh.2013.115

[154] Ercolini D, Fogliano V. Food Design To Feed the Human Gut Microbiota. *J Agric Food Chem.* 2018;66(15):3754–3758. doi:10.1021/acs.jafc.8b00456

[155] Simmen B, et al. Primate energy input and the evolutionary transition to energy-dense diets in humans. *Proceedings of the Royal Society B: Biological Sciences*. 2017;284(1856):20170577. doi:10.1098/rspb.2017.0577.

[156] Meydani SN, Das SK, Pieper CF, et al. Long-term moderate calorie restriction inhibits inflammation without impairing cell-mediated immunity: a randomized controlled trial in non-obese humans. *Aging (Albany NY).* 2016;8(7):1416–1431. doi:10.18632/aging.100994

[157] Sun Y, Liu B, Du Y, et al. Inverse Association between Organic Food Purchase and Diabetes Mellitus in US Adults. *Nutrients*. 2018;10(12):1877. Published 2018 Dec 3. doi:10.3390/nu10121877

[158]https://d2ouvy59p0dg6k.cloudfront.net/downloads/plastic_ingestion_web_spreads.pdf

[159]https://www.nal.usda.gov/afsic/organic

[160]Mie A, Andersen HR, Gunnarsson S, et al. Human health implications of organic food and organic agriculture: a comprehensive review. *Environmental Health*. 2017;16:111. doi:10.1186/s12940-017-0315-4.

[161] Hyland C, Bradman A, Gerona R, Patton S, Zakharevich I, Gunier RB, Klein K. Organic diet intervention significantly reduces urinary pesticide levels in U.S. children and adults. Environ Res. 2019 Apr;171:568-575. doi: 10.1016/j.envres.2019.01.024. Epub 2019 Feb 12.

[162] Yang T, Doherty J, Zhao B, Kinchla AJ, Clark JM, He L. Effectiveness of

Commercial and Homemade Washing Agents in Removing Pesticide Residues on and in Apples. J Agric Food Chem. 2017 Nov 8;65(44):9744-9752. doi: 10.1021/acs.jafc.7b03118. Epub 2017 Oct 25.

[163]Furmli S, Elmasry R, Ramos M, Fung J. Therapeutic use of intermittent fasting for people with type 2 diabetes as an alternative to insulin. *BMJ Case Rep.* 2018;2018:bcr2017221854. Published 2018 Oct 9. doi:10.1136/bcr-2017-221854

[164] Gabel K, Hoddy KK, Haggerty N, et al. Effects of 8-hour time restricted feeding on body weight and metabolic disease risk factors in obese adults: A pilot study. *Nutr Healthy Aging.* 2018;4(4):345–353. Published 2018 Jun 15. doi:10.3233/NHA-170036

[165] Mitchell SJ, Bernier M, Mattison JA, Aon MA, Kaiser TA, Anson RM, Ikeno Y, Anderson RM, Ingram DK, de Cabo R. Daily Fasting Improves Health and Survival in Male Mice Independent of Diet Composition and Calories. Cell Metab. 2019 Jan 8;29(1):221-228.e3. doi: 10.1016/j.cmet.2018.08.011. Epub 2018 Sep 6.

[166] DiNicolantonio JJ, McCarty M. Autophagy-induced degradation of Notch1, achieved through intermittent fasting, may promote beta cell neogenesis: implications for reversal of type 2 diabetes. *Open Heart.* 2019;6(1):e001028. Published 2019 May 22. doi:10.1136/openhrt-2019-001028

[167] Zhang S, Ratliff EP, Molina B, et al. Aging and Intermittent Fasting Impact on Transcriptional Regulation and Physiological Responses of Adult Drosophila Neuronal and Muscle Tissues. *Int J Mol Sci.* 2018;19(4):1140. Published 2018 Apr 10. doi:10.3390/ijms19041140

[168]Ganesan K, Habboush Y, Sultan S. Intermittent Fasting: The Choice for a Healthier Lifestyle. *Cureus.* 2018;10(7):e2947. Published 2018 Jul 9. doi:10.7759/cureus.2947

[169]Cioffi I, Evangelista A, Ponzo V, et al. Intermittent versus continuous energy restriction on weight loss and cardiometabolic outcomes: a systematic review and meta-analysis of randomized controlled trials. *J Transl Med.* 2018;16(1):371. Published 2018 Dec 24. doi:10.1186/s12967-018-1748-4

[170]Lashinger LM, O'Flanagan CH, Dunlap SM, et al. Starving cancer from the outside and inside: separate and combined effects of calorie restriction and autophagy inhibition on Ras-driven tumors. *Cancer Metab.* 2016;4:18. Published 2016 Sep 16. doi:10.1186/s40170-016-0158-4

[171] Vasto S, Rizzo C, Caruso C. Centenarians and diet: what they eat in the Western part of Sicily. *Immun Ageing*. 2012;9(1):10. Published 2012 Apr 23. doi:10.1186/1742-4933-9-10

[172] You can use this website to see the nutritional breakdown of any food, including plants, meats, etc.: https://fdc.nal.usda.gov/index.html

[173] Antunes F, Erustes AG, Costa AJ, et al. Autophagy and intermittent fasting: the connection for cancer therapy?. *Clinics (Sao Paulo)*. 2018;73(suppl 1):e814s. Published 2018 Dec 10. doi:10.6061/clinics/2018/e814s

[174]Schwartsburd PM. Catabolic and anabolic faces of insulin resistance and their disorders: a new insight into circadian control of metabolic disorders leading to diabetes. *Future Science OA*. 2017;3(3):FSO201. doi:10.4155/fsoa-2017-0015.

[175] Yuan T, Huang X, Woodcock M, et al. Plasma extracellular RNA profiles in healthy and cancer patients. *Sci Rep*. 2016;6:19413. Published 2016 Jan 20. doi:10.1038/srep19413

[176] Olshansky SJ, Rattan SI. What determines longevity: Metabolic rate or stability? Discov Med. 2005 Aug;5(28):359-62.

[177] Galgani J, Ravussin E. Energy metabolism, fuel selection and body weight regulation. *Int J Obes (Lond)*. 2008;32 Suppl 7(Suppl 7):S109–S119. doi:10.1038/ijo.2008.246

[178] Higgins JA. Whole grains, legumes, and the subsequent meal effect: implications for blood glucose control and the role of fermentation. *J Nutr Metab*. 2012;2012:829238. doi:10.1155/2012/829238

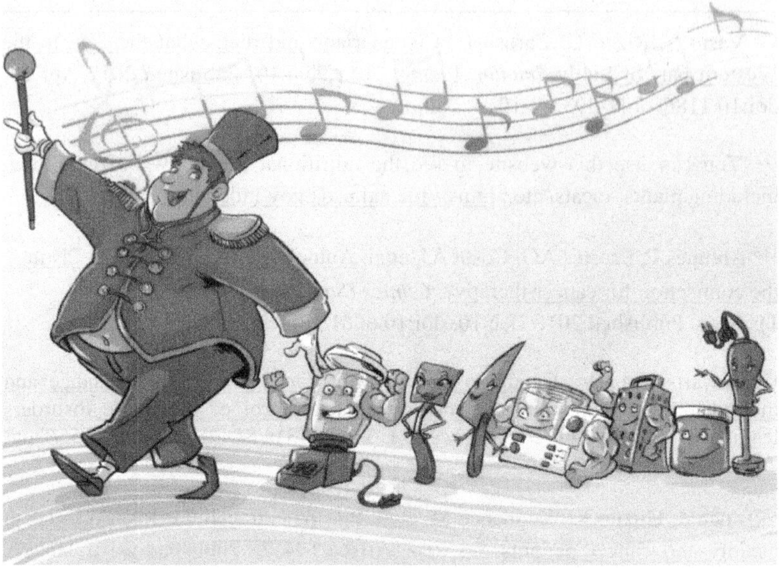

CHAPTER 4

SIMPLE BUT WITH A LITTLE DASH OF EFFORT

Now let's put the Wash Cycle Diet to plate.

I know what many of you are thinking: I don't want to eat raw salads all day. Don't worry. In this chapter, I will show you many ways to make raw food consumption exciting and tasty. Keep in mind that no amount of sugar, cholesterol, animal protein, or fried food is worth the memory loss, arthritic pain, or severe bouts of heartburn and stomach pain around the corner if you don't get your act together now.

The first couple of weeks on the Wash Cycle Diet will be the toughest because of the massive adjustments you have to make. You will not be able to stop and grab a candy bar or a slice of pizza on the fly at a gas station, or a quick meal at a fast-food joint. Unless you live in a metropolitan area that has raw restaurants, your menu choices will be seriously limited. You will have to stop drinking alcohol and smoking cigarettes. These are BIG adjustments, and you will have withdrawal just like all addicts. It will not be easy to just change your diet from cold turkey because there are simply no raw foods that will give you the prolonged feeling of satisfaction like a Western meal. The desire for alcohol, drugs, and processed food products will be hard to manage. When you change your diet for a week or so, your body will start to reverse these feelings of addiction.

My goal here is to help you avoid the trial and error that would discourage many from following through. There is an old saying: give someone a fish and you feed them for a day, teach them to fish and you feed them for a lifetime. There are two big obstacles ahead of you: not having the right tools and a lack of knowledge about food choices. There are dozens of cookbooks out there that promote some version of a raw diet. I have probably read all of them. If you peruse through a raw book and see that they use oils, sugar, syrups, or flour; or the book is filled with recipes that use olive, avocado, or coconut oil; or cauliflower, almond, or coconut flour; or large quantities of sugary syrups like maple or honey, don't waste your time. When you process almonds and coconuts down to flour or use oil from olives or coconuts, or you add half a cup of date/maple syrup or honey, you are no longer following the diet. Also, before you buy any cookbooks, view some of the videos linked on our website (rawrevolution.biz). These videos will give you the visual "how-to" you need to imagine successful raw dishes.

TOOLS YOU NEED

There are a handful of gadgets you need in your raw kitchen. The main appliances in a raw kitchen are a high-speed blender, food processor, and dehydrator.

> ►The blender should be an emulsifying blender. It should have a big motor. Also, make sure it has a tamper so you can mash things down. Some brands will overheat easily, so look at the reviews carefully. The highest price is not necessarily the best product.
>
> ►You will also need a powerful food processor. Some of the butter nut-heavy desserts, sweetened with raw dates, can challenge food processors with weak motors.
>
> ►You will also need a dehydrator. Make sure you buy a large unit with several trays and nonstick dehydrator sheets. The ideal temperature range for us is between 105° and 120°F for a duration of twenty-four hours.

You will also want some other tools in your kitchen: a spiralizer, hand chopper, corn stripper, slicer, strainers, zester, and spatulas. Mason jars with large mouths are great to keep sauces and dressings fresh for a day or two in the refrigerator.

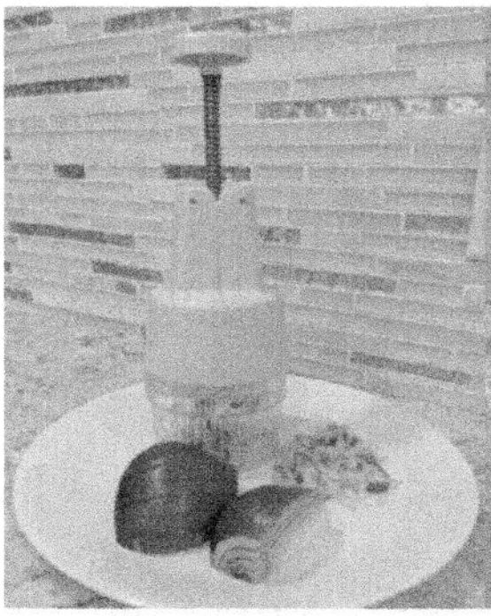
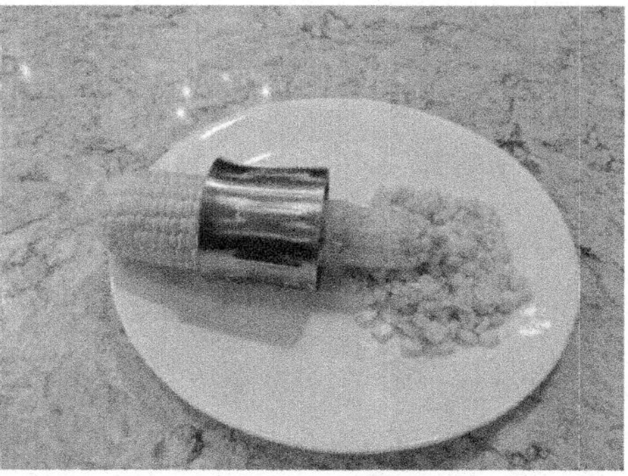
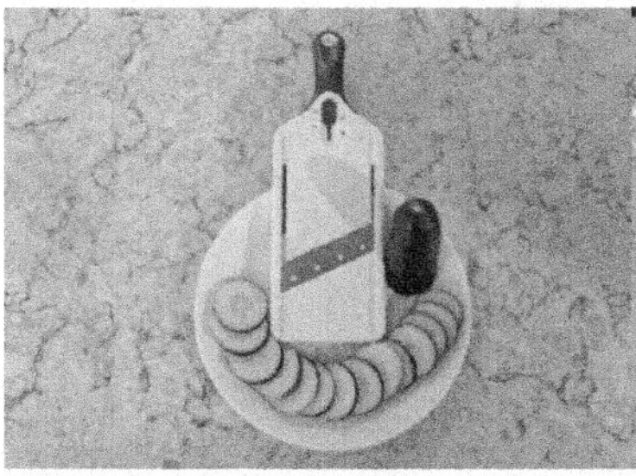
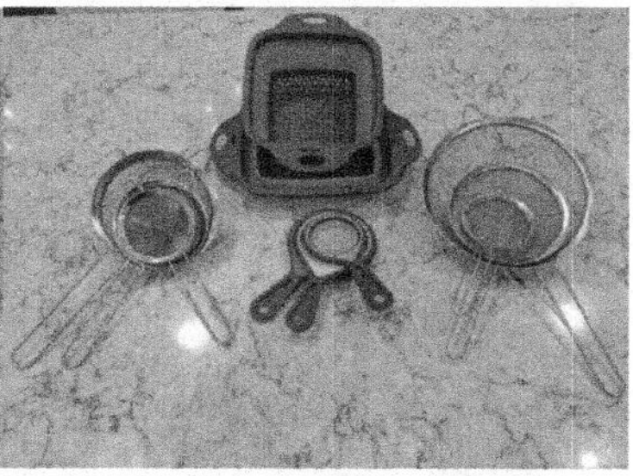
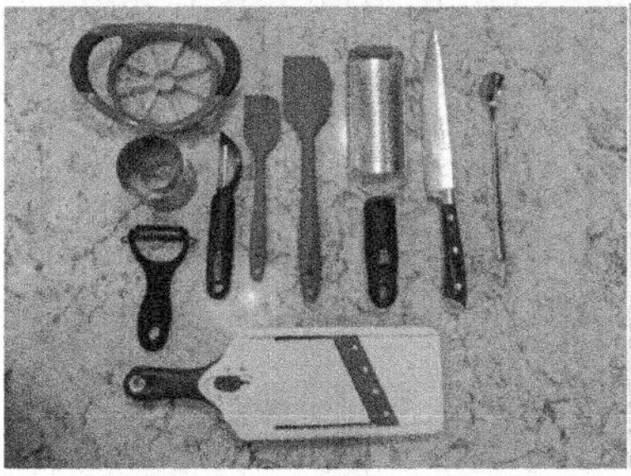
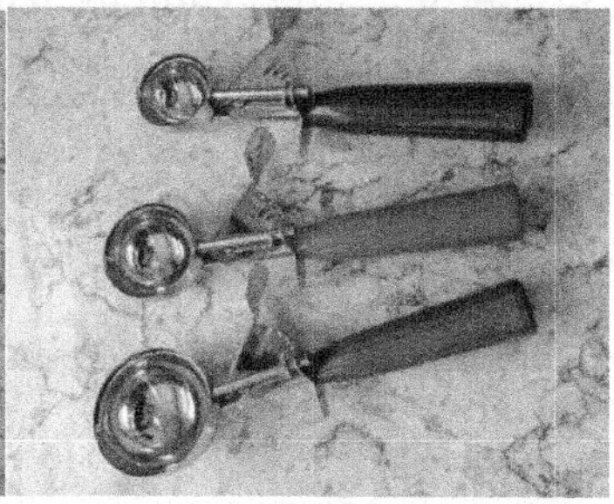
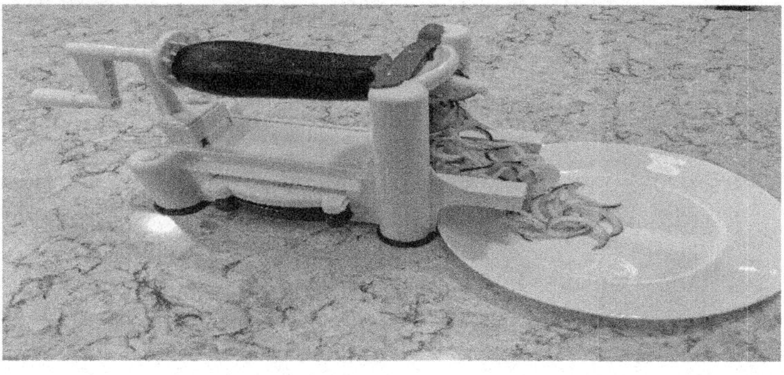

What you eat from now on will be uncooked and unprocessed. The only exception is legumes (beans), which must be cooked to be edible. If whole raw plants remain 80% of what you eat, the other 20% of your daily diet can be emulsified raw ingredients or cooked beans. An example is a dish of raw sliced vegetables (80%) with a dipping sauce made from hummus free of oil and sugar (20%). A food processor/emulsifying blender will break down what you eat to some extent, but even after a minute or two in these mastic blenders, raw food still retains much of its cellular fiber and structure.

Buying Raw Foods

When you shop raw, you must pay close attention to what you buy. For example, banana chips may look healthy and safe to eat, but these chips are usually fried in oil and sweetened. Many dried fruits are soaked in sugar and dried sweet. Some places use high temperature drying and sometimes dried fruits and vegetables are roasted and even fried. The same goes for many nut assortments. They are usually roasted. You may pick a seemingly safe trail mix off the shelf, but it may very well break the rules of the Wash Cycle Diet.

Also, read the labels of anything you buy that is packaged, canned, or jarred. A label that says "natural" really means nothing. If a seller could say free of synthetic chemicals or pesticides on its label, it would. Store-bought peanut or almond butter is usually roasted and sweetened. Pay attention to the fat and sugar content of the label and make sure there is no added oil or sugar, that there is no roasting, and that you steer clear of as many synthetic chemicals as possible. Even when you go to the farmers' market, there is no guarantee that anything you buy is free of pesticides or synthetic chemicals. Keep in mind that although you can't wash synthetic pesticides off fruits and vegetables, you can neutralize the pesticides sprayed on conventional raw plants by soaking fruits and vegetables in an alkalizing agent, such as sodium bicarbonate (baking soda) water mixture, for fifteen minutes.

Your diet will become dependent on which fruits, vegetables, and edible plants are available fresh at your supermarket. Whether you live in Florida or Maine, fruits are generally grown in certain warm climates all year long or in a greenhouse and shipped across the country. Generally, there will be access to apples, bananas, melons, oranges, and grapes year-round, but things like pomegranate, nectarines, peaches, or cherries might be difficult to find at certain times of the year. The same goes for vegetables. Carrots, cauliflower, broccoli, cucumbers, celery, lettuce, peppers, zucchini, and squash are around all year, but more exotic squashes, string beans, or some leafy greens may only be available at certain times of the year or only frozen. Many grocery stores do have decent selections of organic frozen berries, fruits, greens, and vegetables, which are acceptable to use. You can also indefinitely store dried spices, nuts, and seeds in bulk, preferably in a dry cool place or in your freezer.

The Base and How to Flavor It

The base of a raw food diet is always fruits, vegetables, greens, nuts, beans, grains, and seeds. You can use the blender, processor, and cooked beans to emulsify a tasty raw-based product that tends to take on a certain taste profile. For example, a dip with a base of peppers can have a tangier taste, whereas carrot and corn tend to be sweet and creamy, celery tends to be salty and fibrous, cashews are savory and creamy, zucchini or squash have more of a fermented flavor, and cooked beans can accent any spice profile. Use the raw produce or beans and just enough water to produce a watery mortar-like consistency in your mastic blender and taste it. Then as you add each additional ingredient, continue to taste your mixture.

Certain flavors are needed to make dressing and dips trigger your happy senses.[179] Just because you eat raw doesn't mean that essential flavor profiles become less important. Most culinary books talk about balancing flavors: sweet, sour (acid), salty, and savory (fatty). These flavors work just as effectively with raw food and can be used to make all sorts of tasty bases, dips, and dressings:

► Sour or acid: vinegar (endless varieties from apple cider to grape, pear, or other balsamic types are all acceptable)[180] and lemon/lime juices.

► Salty: sea salts loaded with minerals are extremely healthy and should be a normal part of your diet. Use Himalayan or Celtic salt but go easy on salt use until your vitals are back to normal (salt is discussed more in the next chapter).[181]

► Sweet: sweetness can come from dates or dried fruits. Dates are my favorite and a major staple of any raw kitchen, and the most flavorful type of date is the Medjool.[182] I go through a small package of dates in as few as two days. Dates are generally free of pesticides and chemicals, so it's up to you if you want to buy certified organic dates. You can also use dried fruits like raisins that can be soaked for an hour to plump up.

► Fatty: blended nuts, hemp seeds, nut butter, and tahini (ground sesame seeds), coconut, almonds, cashews, avocadoes, and olives can be used in dressings, hummus, and desserts to bring that savory, fatty flavor in place of oils, butter, lard, eggs, and dairy.

Raw food dishes can have many different flavors, such as Asian or Middle Eastern. By using nutritional yeast, you can add a cheesy/nutty flavor. Things like dulce (seaweed), soy sauce, and raw miso can provide Asian flavors. Some smoked paprika, sun-dried tomatoes, or chili paste can give a Mexican/Spanish taste. Garlic, cumin, or turmeric with some fresh olives can add a Middle Eastern flare. Cinnamon and cacao can add sweet aromas and flavor. Mustard is a super tangy all-around flavor enhancer. Raw butter such as almond butter, peanut butter, and tahini are excellent replacements for oil and fats. Cooked beans, peas, and corn can serve as ingredients for your dressings or as garnishes or fillers. Corn and string beans are perfectly edible raw but most other beans must be cooked or they can be toxic.[183]

When it comes to flavor enhancers, the amount you will use is a small percentage of any meal (5% or so), so don't worry about raw purity to achieve flavor. I use reduced vegetable or chili bouillons for deeper flavors and a company called Better Than Bouillon® makes great ones. You have a busy life, so don't turn food preparation into something that gives you anxiety or that requires you to waste time shopping or preparing.

FRUITS

Fruits should become a major part of your diet.[184] Some folks criticize raw eaters, calling them *fruitaholics* for eating large amounts of sugary fruits. This is pure nonsense. A seven-year study looking at half a million people in China found that "higher fresh fruit consumption was associated with significantly lower risk of diabetes".[185] Raw sugary fruits, such as a date, will not cause your blood sugar to spike uncontrollably.[186] There are days I have eaten a dozen dates and the effect is gradual and managed. It takes a lot of effort for your body to extract the complex sugars found in fruits and you will not digest a high percentage of the simple sugars in fruits because of your body's inability to extract them from the fibers it is bound to.[187]

You can eat all the fruits you want on the Wash Cycle diet. This is true especially during the first two weeks of the diet. The fruits overload will help replace the feeling you used to get from processed foods and sugar. Fruits like sweet grapes, very sweet watermelon, or overripe bananas will combat the withdrawal symptoms from a Western diet.[188] Eat all the ripe bananas,[189] berries,[190] grapes,[191] blueberries,[192] cantaloupes, peaches, and apricots,[193] as fruits are filled with antioxidants and plant power.

In today's supermarkets, you will without a doubt be disappointed with the ripeness of most fruits sold. The fruit industry has waged a 50-year war against ethylene, the molecular compound responsible for fruit ripening.[194] All sorts of supposedly edible synthetic chemicals have been developed to prolong the shelf life of fruit[195] in the name of efficiency and profit, and at the expense of your health. Smell your fruit. Give it a squeeze. Every piece of fruit should have an aroma and be slightly soft to the touch. Watermelons should have a hollow knock. Cantaloupes and honey melons should smell sweet. If the fruit leaves a white film on you, don't buy it. Be sure to peel citrus fruits completely as many are painted with spray plastics.

NUTS AND HIGH-FAT PLANTS

The fat in nuts, avocados, olives, coconuts, chia and flax seeds, and other plants are extremely healthy for you in raw form.[196] You can soak chia seeds for a few hours to make puddings or desserts. Flax seeds can be used to build a base for dehydrated crackers. Nuts, coconuts, avocados, or olives can replace the savory taste of meats, cheeses, and oil. High-fat raw nuts and fruits have many applications in raw cuisine.

There are five nuts/seeds that are commonly available at your grocery/health food store: almonds, cashews, hemp, walnuts, and sunflowers.[197] Raw cashews and hulled hemp are soft and can be used in place of oil or cream in your mastic blender to give a savory taste. You can soak raw cashews for fifteen minutes and they will start to get squishy. Walnuts and almonds tend to be harder and are more edible raw when soaked overnight and better suited for dessert bases. Sunflower seeds are easy to work with and make a great hearty base chopped up in a food processor. These nuts and seeds are relatively inexpensive compared to the price of meat and can be found easily in raw and even raw organic form. Sometimes you may even find these nuts *unpasteurized*, which some on the extreme side may strive for so as not to degrade the nutritional value of the produce.[198]

If you have ever bought any kind of nut butter, you will notice that the oil separates out. This extra oil is *why* you can use nuts and nut butter as oil replacement. This same oil is also why you cannot use large portions of this butter. Plant milk like coconut milk and nut butter are in a middle sort of no man's land when it comes to the Wash Cycle Diet because of the level of processing it takes to make milk or butter, and although you can use them, they should be used in moderation. When you make a dressing, use a spoon or two of plant milk or nut butter, not a can or several scoops. Tahini (sesame paste) is another healthy regular oil replacement that can be used to make hummus. Coconut milk can be bought in milky or creamy consistency.

Although studies have shown no major effect on blood fat levels with increased consumption of plant milk[199] and nut butter, they should still be used in moderation during the Wash Cycle Diet so you can achieve the level of autophagy required. Once the Wash Cycle Diet is over, you can indulge more regularly in these nut butters and milks.

Salads, Dips, and Dressings

The staple of your diet will be an uncooked dish of various mixtures of raw greens, vegetables, fruits, nuts, and/or some cooked legumes. Use beans, vegetables, fruits, raw overnight soaked nuts, and seeds to make vibrant salads. You can add sprouts like alfalfa, broccoli, or mung bean. With the right dressing flavors, you will never grow tired of what we globally call salad.

Since your base is going to be fruits and vegetables, the most important flavor component to your meal will be the dressing or dip you make. Virtually all commercial salad dressings are loaded with oil and sugar. Even when you consume just a few tablespoons of conventional dressing, the oil and sugar content in the dressing will make it difficult to meet the strict requirements of the Wash Cycle Diet. A cup of commercial dressing contains about half a cup of oil and a quarter cup of sugar. By taking out the processed oil and sugar content found in conventional dressings, you take in a neutral or negative number of digestible calories, even if you eat two or three pounds of raw fruits and vegetables for a meal. When making dressings, use sweeter vegetables like corn, carrot, dates, nuts, nut butter, or coconut milk as bases in your dressing so that the dressing is sweeter and more savory. Dressing can be simple yet delicious. Here is a very simple but tasty dressing celery-based dressing:

- ► Three or four stalks of celery
- ► ¼ cup of tahini
- ► A couple of dates
- ► Lemon juice, sea salt, and water to taste.

You can make a corn-based dressing:

- ► One cup fresh corn
- ► ¼ cup coconut milk
- ► Dates to taste
- ► Smoked paprika, salt, apple cider vinegar to taste
- ► Water until you have the right consistency
- ► Mix an additional 1/3 cup of corn to the final product

Another choice can be a chipotle-style dressing:

- ► One cup cashews
- ► Smaller whole tomato
- ► ¼ cup of black beans
- ► Better Than Bouillon® Chili base to taste
- ► Smoked paprika, salt, vinegar (balsamic) to taste
- ► Water until you have the right consistency
- ► Mix in another ¼ cup of whole black beans

Another choice is a Caesar-style dressing:

- ► ½ cup unsweetened almond milk
- ► One cup of cashews
- ► ¼ cup of nutritional yeast
- ► Dates, Dijon mustard to taste
- ► Lemon juice, soy sauce, salt, and pepper to taste
- ► Water until you have the desired consistency

These dressings can be just as decadent, and savory as comparable ones made from oil and sugar. Taste your dressing after every ingredient you add. To make things even more savory, you can use nut butter or coconut milk. If it seems a little low on sugar, add a date. Not sour enough? Add a little more lemon juice, apple cider, or balsamic vinegar. Nutritional yeast will provide a cheesy flavor. Sprinkle a little extra sea salt for a saltier taste. Soy sauce or miso is great for Asian flavors. Dulce (seaweed) gives a fishy flavor. Vegetable bullion or chili bases add deep flavors. Always have a little extra water handy so you can alter the consistency.

We can easily replace oil and sugar, and by using a mastic blender, the result is a healthy and tasty alternative that does not have a lot of easily digestible calories yet still tastes great. Your dressing can have a fruit base, vegetable base, or a nut base (or a mixture). Try different raw ingredients and as you taste the mix, compare the salt, sweet, sour, and savory flavors to find a good balance. Make small amounts and if it strikes you as tasty, store the recipe in a place you can access again and again, and make larger quantities you can store in a mason jar that can hold for an additional day or two.

A favorite dip for me is hummus. A ton of oil is added to commercially produced hummus (one of the top three ingredients). The key is to replace this oil with tahini, and the beans, even though cooked and blended, still require significant work to digest,[200] are very tasty, easy to make, and super healthy.[201]

The basic hummus recipe is essentially cooked chickpeas (garbanzo beans) ground up in a blender. Cut up some carrots, cauliflower, broccoli, or bell peppers to dip into the hummus:

- One cup of organic chickpeas
- ¼ medium-sized red onion
- ½ cup tahini
- Dates and garlic to taste
- Himalayan salt and pepper to taste
- Lemon juice to taste
- Water until you have the right consistency

Your salad can range from a traditional salad to a cabbage-based coleslaw-style salad, a kale-based salad, or even a broccoli and cauliflower salad. Add finely chopped radishes, carrots, water chestnuts, fruit, baby corn, green peppers, or beans. Here are some quick salad ideas:

- Berry pear salad w/red wine poppy seed dressing
- Orange sesame Asian salad
- Broccoli salad
- Mexican corn salad
- Creamy cucumber salad
- Cucumber and melon salad w/Dijon dressing
- Mango and avocado salad

Crackers and Wraps

Crackers and wraps are excellent replacements for bread. Dip these in hummus or other dips you make or eat with the salad or soup you prepared. Use them as bread for comfort foods, or as wraps for raw burritos. These are super easy to make. Here is a vegetable cracker recipe using an emulsifying blender:

►Put a cut-up onion in the blender and add water so it covers the onion. Pulse until the onion is in little bitty pieces. Drain in a fine strainer to remove the water. Do the same with two cut carrots and two celery stalks.

►Add flax seeds, garlic paste, lemon juice, and soy sauce to taste.

► Combine everything and mix by hand until you have the consistency of mortar. Use dehydrator sheets and spread the mix up to 1/2-to-3/4-inch thickness onto the sheets. Use a knife to make lines for easy cracker sizes later. Dehydrate for 12 hours at 115°. Flip. Dehydrate for another 8-12 hours at 115° until you have a crunchy consistency.

To make a wrap using the dehydrator, add a bit more water to the mixture, lay it thinner, and dehydrate at 105° instead of 115°. You can even make sweet wraps with fruit, dates, and chia seeds. You need to pre-plan for wraps and crackers. I have a nine-drawer dehydrator that can make enough to last for a few days. Also, I generally tend to use my stale vegetables as part of the base to use them up. If you decide to make large quantities, make sure you have extra-large metal bowls, a large but fine strainer, and strong mixing spatulas with a long, thick handle.

SOUPS

If you dilute beans/carrots/corn with some extra water in your blender for several minutes, you will get a warm soup because an emulsifying blender will heat things up. Add some room temperature finely diced tomatoes, diced green onions, some whole black beans, season to taste, and you have a warm black bean soup or vegetarian oil-free chili. Your high-speed blender will warm food and get it right up to 115°F if you so desire, and you still have not ultra-processed any part of what you made. You can also take the drawers out of your large dehydrator and warm the soups or any other fake comfort food for an hour or so to give it a chance to bind itself better. Add some dehydrated crackers and you have a fantastic meal.

PUDDINGS, SNACKS, SMOOTHIES, AND DESSERTS

Raw food can be adapted to make all sorts of treats and desserts as well. You can soak Chia seeds overnight and the result is a pudding consistency. After a long soaking, add some fruit, coconut, cacao, carob, nuts, and/or seeds. An easy breakfast favorite is ½ cup of Chia seeds soaked overnight. Add a bit of coconut milk to give it a creamy consistency. Then add some sweet fruit.

When you get hungry for a snack, you can snack on nuts and dried fruit medleys bought at stores, or just soak some raw walnuts or almonds overnight in water, which will soften them, so they are delicious to eat raw even if you don't have the best teeth. One of my favorites is a medley of raw pumpkin seeds, cashews, walnuts, dried mulberries, red and golden raisins, goji berries, currants, and cacao nibs.

You can also make a smoothie. Sweet watermelons, ripe mangos, grapes, cherries, and berries may or may not be available in your region during certain times of the year, but you can access organic and unpreserved frozen fruits all year round. I can usually readily find organic frozen cherries, mangoes, strawberries, raspberries, and blueberries even at big chain stores. I add a heavy dose of dates because I like my smoothie sweet. I usually will have a smoothie as my first food of the day. I also add some additional plant ingredients which we will discuss in much more detail in the next chapter.

Finally, you will crave an occasional treat. The easiest things to make are very similar to the energy bars you get at the store, but with raw ingredients, and usually shaped into balls. Overindulgence on power bar type desserts will push the limits of a calorie neutral/negative diet, although nothing made raw comes close to the sugar, flour, and oil content found in a candy bar. I have a sweet tooth, so I don't mind a daily indulgence with some green tea. These treats are very easy to make. Take one cup of almonds and process them in a food processor until they are finely chopped. Add ½ cup of almond butter, 1/4 cup of carob powder, 1/4 cup or more of fresh soft dates, and a dash of vanilla extract. Mix and masticate the dry ingredients before you add the butter and dates. Let the mixture blend well, clump, and once you have a mortar consistency, roll chunks into a ball. Take some almonds soaked over the night before and push them into the ball with your thumb until secure. Place in the refrigerator or freezer for one to three hours until firm.

Another regular treat for me is sunflower based. Place a cup of sunflower seeds in the food processor and break the seeds down finely. Then add about ½ cup of tahini and a ½ cup of dates. Garnish with previously soaked walnuts or even some coconut dust. Place in the refrigerator or freezer for one to three hours until firm, and then cut into small pieces. These are great for when you get that urge for something sweet and savory. These desserts have high contents of good fats and are sweetened naturally.

COMFORT FOODS

Many of the Western food products we eat can be recreated by using some imagination with raw food. Take any conventional recipe and break down its ingredients. There is always a base or filler, and then look for the flavors added to make the dish special. In virtually every instance, there is a raw replacement you can use to get a delicious equivalent.

Let's take the traditional spaghetti and meatballs. Use spiral vegetables instead of pasta. Use an emulsifying blender to make the sauce. For a Southwestern marinara-type sauce, combine two cups of tomatoes, two bell peppers, basil, balsamic vinegar, a red onion, some tomato paste, and a clove of garlic with water in the blender. Instead of cooked ground meat, oil, and flour to make meatballs, blend walnuts and mushrooms with some herbs and lemon juice until you have a clumpy mixture, dehydrate at 115° for six hours (or until firm), and you have spaghetti and meatballs with marinara sauce!

How about macaroni and cheese? Use spiraled vegetables like squash or zucchini as macaroni. Simulate the cheese by mixing two cups of cashews, 1/2 cup of nutritional yeast, water, lemon juice, garlic, and half an onion in a blender until you have a sauce consistency. Pour over the spirals and add salt and pepper to taste. Warm it in the dehydrator for an hour at 115°.

How about a fake tuna salad? Use a blender to crush sunflower seeds, add some lemon juice, finely chopped celery, and some dulce (seaweed) to get the fishy flavor, and add herbs, spices, salt, and pepper to taste, and you have a very respectable fishy-tasting tuna salad. Put the fake tuna on your dehydrated crackers and eat as many as you like until you get that satisfied feeling.

How about an Asian-flavored bowl of noodles and sauce? Use the longer spiral option on your spiralizer to spiral vegetables that look like pasta for noodles. Take 1/2 cup of almond butter, one chopped red onion, two stalks of green onion, two tablespoons of soy sauce, one tablespoon of miso, some ginger, garlic, three to four dates, one tablespoon of vegetable bouillon base, and some water and blend until you get the right consistency (just above liquid). For a pastier consistency, you can also add some tahini (sesame paste). If you want some sweetness, add a few dates. Warm it in the dehydrator for an hour at 115°.

Take any original recipe, find alternatives, and use the high-speed blender, the chopper, and a dehydrator, and you can make anything raw, without processed meats, eggs, dairy, oil, flour, and sugar.

WHERE TO FIND RAW RECIPES

There are lots of free recipes from raw food enthusiasts brought together with links on our website for your viewing pleasure (rawrevolution.biz). Many people out there have shared their knowledge online.

---

[179]Chaudhari N, Roper SD. The cell biology of taste. *The Journal of Cell Biology*. 2010;190(3):285-296. doi:10.1083/jcb.201003144.

[180]Mitrou P, Petsiou E, Papakonstantinou E, et al. Vinegar Consumption Increases Insulin-Stimulated Glucose Uptake by the Forearm Muscle in Humans with Type 2 Diabetes. *Journal of Diabetes Research*. 2015;2015:175204.

[181] Lee BH, Yang AR, Kim MY, McCurdy S, Boisvert WA. Natural sea salt consumption confers protection against hypertension and kidney damage in Dahl salt-sensitive rats. 2017 Mar 20;61(1):1300375]. *Food Nutr Res*. 2016;61(1):1264713. Published 2016 Dec 20.

[182] Al-Shahib W, Marshall RJ. The fruit of the date palm: its possible use as the best food for the future? Int J Food Sci Nutr. 2003 Jul;54(4):247-59. Review.

[183] Nciri N, Cho N. New research highlights: Impact of chronic ingestion of white kidney beans (*Phaseolus vulgaris* L. var. Beldia) on small-intestinal disaccharidase activity in Wistar rats. *Toxicol Rep*. 2017;5:46–55. Published 2017 Dec 15. doi:10.1016/j.toxrep.2017.12.016

[184]Dreher ML. Whole Fruits and Fruit Fiber Emerging Health Effects. *Nutrients*. 2018;10(12):1833. Published 2018 Nov 28. doi:10.3390/nu10121833

[185]Du H, Li L, Bennett D, et al. Fresh fruit consumption in relation to incident diabetes and diabetic vascular complications: A 7-y prospective study of 0.5 million Chinese adults. *PLoS Med*. 2017;14(4):e1002279. Published 2017 Apr 11. doi:10.1371/journal.pmed.1002279

[186]Alkaabi JM, Al-Dabbagh B, Ahmad S, Saadi HF, Gariballa S, Ghazali MA.

Glycemic indices of five varieties of dates in healthy and diabetic subjects. *Nutr J.* 2011;10:59. Published 2011 May 28. doi:10.1186/1475-2891-10-59

[187] Sharma SP, Chung HJ, Kim HJ, Hong ST. Paradoxical Effects of Fruit on Obesity. *Nutrients.* 2016;8(10):633. Published 2016 Oct 14. doi:10.3390/nu8100633

[188] Wang PY, Fang JC, Gao ZH, Zhang C, Xie SY. Higher intake of fruits, vegetables or their fiber reduces the risk of type 2 diabetes: A meta-analysis. *J Diabetes Investig.* 2016;7(1):56–69. doi:10.1111/jdi.12376

[189]Adedayo BC, Oboh G, Oyeleye SI, OlasehindeTA.Antioxidant and Antihyperglycemic Properties of Three Banana Cultivars (*Musa* spp.). *Scientifica (Cairo).* 2016;2016:8391398. doi:10.1155/2016/8391398

[190]Vendrame S, Del Bo' C, Ciappellano S, Riso P, Klimis-Zacas D. Berry Fruit Consumption and Metabolic Syndrome. *Antioxidants (Basel).* 2016;5(4):34. Published 2016 Sep 30. doi:10.3390/antiox5040034

[191]Testa R, Bonfigli AR, Genovese S, De Nigris V, Ceriello A. The Possible Role of Flavonoids in the Prevention of Diabetic Complications. *Nutrients.* 2016;8(5):310. Published 2016 May 20. doi:10.3390/nu8050310

[192]Stull AJ.Blueberries' Impact on Insulin Resistance and Glucose Intolerance. *Antioxidants (Basel).* 2016;5(4):44. Published 2016 Nov 29. doi:10.3390/antiox5040044

[193]Xu H, Luo J, Huang J, Wen Q. Flavonoids intake and risk of type 2 diabetes mellitus: A meta-analysis of prospective cohort studies. *Medicine (Baltimore).* 2018;97(19):e0686. doi:10.1097/MD.0000000000010686

[194]Burg SP, Burg EA. Role of Ethylene in Fruit Ripening. *Plant Physiol.* 1962;37(2):179–189. doi:10.1104/pp.37.2.179

[195]Dave RK, Ramana Rao TV, Nandane AS. Improvement of post-harvest quality of pear fruit with optimized composite edible coating formulations. *J Food Sci Technol.* 2017;54(12):3917–3927. doi:10.1007/s13197-017-2850-y

[196]Hernández-Alonso P, Camacho-Barcia L, Bulló M, Salas-Salvadó J. Nuts and Dried Fruits: An Update of Their Beneficial Effects on Type 2 Diabetes. *Nutrients.* 2017;9(7):673. Published 2017 Jun 28. doi:10.3390/nu9070673

[197]Ros E. Health Benefits of Nut Consumption. *Nutrients*. 2010;2(7):652-682. doi:10.3390/nu2070652.

[198] Aamir M, Ovissipour M, Sablani SS, Rasco B. Predicting the Quality of Pasteurized Vegetables Using Kinetic Models: A Review. *Int J Food Sci*. 2013;2013:271271. doi:10.1155/2013/271271

[199] Ekanayaka RA, Ekanayaka NK, Perera B, De Silva PG. Impact of a traditional dietary supplement with coconut milk and soya milk on the lipid profile in normal free living subjects. *J Nutr Metab*. 2013;2013:481068. doi:10.1155/2013/481068

[200]Thorne M.J., Thompson L.U., Jenkins D.J. Factors affecting starch digestibility and the glycemic response with special reference to legumes. Am. J. Clin. Nutr. 1983;38:481–488.

[201]Wallace TC, Murray R, Zelman KM.The Nutritional Value and Health Benefits of Chickpeas and Hummus. *Nutrients*. 2016;8(12):766. doi:10.3390/nu8120766.

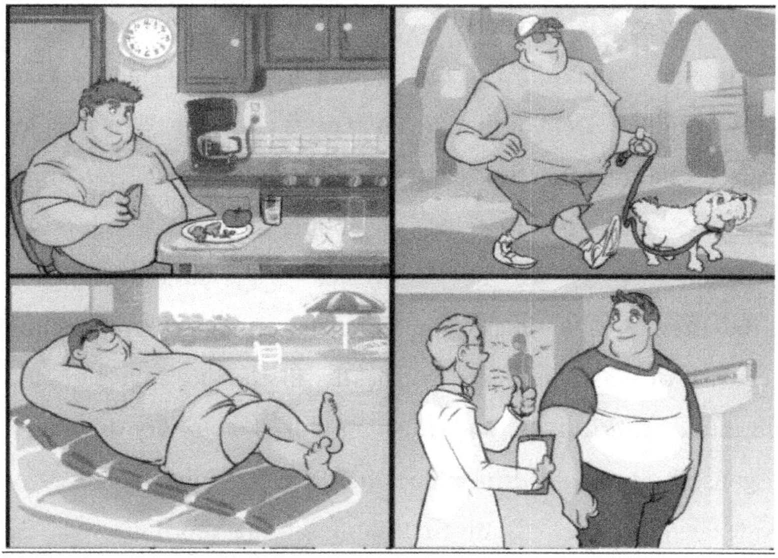

CHAPTER 5

THE TWEAKS OF LIFE

In addition to diet modification, there are certain lifestyle changes that will help you get your body back into top metabolic shape. The goal is to optimize fatty tissue metabolism, improve insulin sensitivity, and reduce oxidative stress that leads to cardiovascular disease, osteoporosis, and sarcopenia (bone and muscle loss). The lifestyle changes in this chapter are specifically tailored to make positive noticeable differences in your health as you age. Incorporate as many of these tweaks as you can.

WATER

The human body is largely made up of water,[202] and as you age, you become much more susceptible to dehydration.[203]

When you get older, your body simply stops telling you that you are thirsty.[204] One-third of our seniors are in a constant state of dehydration.[205] Dehydration, even at minimal levels,[206] is a major cause of inflammation and cognitive decline.[207] Without adequate amounts of water, metabolic dysfunction increases exponentially as we age.[208] Water is essential for good circulation, lymphatic flow, maintenance of body temperature, removal of waste products from cells, facilitating ingestion and digestion, lubrication, and flushing out the urinary tract and organs. You should drink about half your weight in ounces of water every day.[209] Start first thing in the morning with 32 ounces of water and keep drinking intermittently throughout the day until about four hours before you are ready to go to bed.

HEAT, SWEAT, AND MOVEMENT

Although everyone knows how to break a sweat and exercise, the focus for an aging diabetic is to clean and clear, without significant wear and tear.[210] Light exercises like walking, cycling, swimming, or any other low-impact exercise thirty minutes a day will be adequate,[211] or you can increase the impact by combining exercise with heat and sun for optimal results. The best time to exercise is within an hour or so after you eat a big meal.[212]

The lungs and the skin are major excretory pathways. Exercise and sweat increase cardiac output, signal the body to make more blood, and the flow of blood gets redistributed to the skin to create a cooling radiator effect. Exercise will compel the lungs to remove excess carbon waste,[213] and sweat is an effective way of excreting toxins that bio-accumulate in our muscles, tissues, and organs.[214] Exercise is very effective at clearing gunk out of the body and brain.[215]

A sauna, or thermotherapy, is also very effective because it heats the core of the body,[216] triggering the production of enzymes and hormones that reduce oxidative stress and inflammation.[217] As the body's core temperature rises, the body feels threatened and releases countermeasures that stimulate metabolism, providing protection. Make sure that you have proper hydration and that you consume adequate amounts of mineral salts so you don't become dehydrated or create an electrolyte imbalance.[218] Studies have shown that using the sauna regularly significantly reduces total cholesterol levels, the incidence of cardiovascular complications, premature death, dementia, and neuro-degeneration.[219]

SLEEP AND THE CIRCADIAN CLOCK

A good night's sleep is one of the most important parts of healthy aging.[220] The body sleeps in stages. First, your heartbeat, breathing, and eye movements slow, and your muscles relax with occasional twitches. During this light sleep, which lasts for a few minutes, your brain waves begin to slow. Eventually, your body temperature drops, and eye movements stop. Your brain starts to relax. This deeper sleep is why you feel refreshed in the morning. You have the lowest heartbeat and breathing during this stage of sleep. Finally, you go into REM

(Rapid Eye Movement) sleep. During REM, breathing increases, heart rate rises, and blood pressure increases. You go back and forth between deep sleep and REM several times during a typical night with increasingly longer, deeper periods of sleep.

Sleep is controlled by circadian and homeostatic processes.[221] Circadian rhythms control the process and homeostasis controls the intensity. Most adults need seven to nine hours of sleep a night. Avoid light from round-the-clock artificial light and televisions because this blue light suppresses melatonin production,[222] resulting in sleep pattern disruptions.[223] A peanut-sized structure deep inside our brains (hypothalamus) controls sleep.[224] Housed within are clusters of cells that control a variety of glands throughout the body responsible for homeostasis and rhythm.[225]

Sleep disruption has significant negative effects on glucose control.[226] If the *sleep debt* is not sufficiently repaid every night, it accumulates and causes metabolic havoc.[227] It is very common to hear older people describe how they function just fine with five hours of sleep. Five hours of sleep at night is considered "severely short sleep".[228] Sleep forms and maintains pathways for learning and memory. The duration and quality of sleep are extremely important because during sleep, the flow of cerebrospinal fluid in the brain increases dramatically, and this is how the brain washes away waste.[229]

Sleep apnea (where the body stops breathing) and insomnia are common among the elderly.[230] When sleeping habits start to change, this is a major indication that unwanted biological changes are occurring inside your body.[231] Insomnia is a sign of major metabolic dysfunction.[232] If you snore or wake up several times during the night, you should consult with a physician right away and request a prescription for a CPAP (Continuous Positive Airway Pressure) machine.

When it's time to sleep, you should have a dark room with walls that will act as sound buffers. If you cannot achieve total darkness, use an eye cover. If you cannot achieve total quiet, use earplugs. Keep the room at a comfortable temperature,[233] and try not to run a loud air conditioner, and don't keep anything on with blue light, like a computer or TV screen. If your mind starts racing, you wake during the night, or you wake up early and are unable to go back to sleep, read or take some melatonin.[234] Eat pistachios during the day, they are an excellent source of natural slow-release melatonin.

MICRONUTRIENTS

About 1% of our diet comes from micronutrients.[235] Over the last several centuries, we have made significant progress in finding vitamins, minerals, and plant compounds that protect our health and help us heal.[236] Although we see ridiculous claims daily about how micronutrients can turn you into a superman, cure cancer, make you invincible, smarter, or stronger, all these claims are false.

There are a few well-studied micronutrients that are worthy of discussion.[237] We have known for many years that vitamin deficiency can cause horrific metabolic diseases like scurvy or rickets.[238] It has also become apparent that excess intake of vitamins and minerals can also have harmful toxic effects.[239] In our case, because raw food is designed to restrict caloric intake through lower digestibility, we need to make sure that as we switch our diet, we continue to get adequate quantities of essential micronutrients.[240] Government bodies have established Recommended Dietary Allowances (RDAs) for micronutrients.[241] For any of the specific vitamins, take the suggested RDA amounts. The information on a supplement bottle will always tell you the RDA percentage contained in a serving size (a pill, capsule, teaspoon, etc.).

Some vitamins are fat-soluble and others are water-soluble. Fat-soluble vitamins can be stored in our fat, but water-soluble vitamins wash away and must be replenished frequently. There are four fat soluble vitamins (A, D, E, K), and nine water soluble vitamins (eight B vitamins and vitamin C). Fat soluble vitamins can be stored long term in fat cells, but water-soluble vitamins must be replenished regularly. We need to pay particular attention to Vitamins B_{12}, C, and D.

Most folks are vitamin D deficient,[242] and rickets happen when children are deficient in vitamin D and results in the development of bowed legs and bad joints. Vitamin D is called the anti-aging vitamin.[243] It regulates the expression of ~900 genes involved in a wide array of physiological functions[244] and helps metabolize cholesterol.[245] Without adequate amounts of vitamin D, there is muscle loss, an unhealthy immune system, and eventual cardiovascular and neurodegenerative diseases.[246] The best way to get this vitamin is to metabolize it using the sun.[247] You can take vitamin D supplements if you don't want to come out of your cave,[248] but vitamin D pills in large doses tend to also increase mineral absorption,[249] which might lead to the development of kidney stones or decrease joint elasticity,[250] or in less obvious ways, by bringing about neck and head tension aches. If you live in an area like I do, where 200 days a year are overcast and 150 days a year are freezing outside, you can use a vitamin D lamp following the manufacturer's recommendations, which should provide an adequate amount of UV light.[251] If you take a supplement, start with no more than 1000 IUs (international units) a day of a combination of D_3 along with some K_2,[252] which helps with absorption.

For humans, meat and dairy are common sources of Vitamin B_{12} (cobalamins) and most herbivores get this vitamin by consuming vegetation tainted by feces. Because vitamin B_{12} is so important in the fight to reduce oxidative stress and to keep anemia at bay,[253] it is essential for aging plant-eaters to consume adequate amounts of this vitamin.[254] Nutritional yeast, a cheesy flavor used in many raw food recipes discussed in the last chapter, is a good food source for B_{12}.[255]

Vitamin C is another crucial vitamin for metabolism. Vitamin C is an excellent antioxidant and free radical scavenger.[256] Vitamin C also triggers genes inside your cells to either get to work,[257] or self-destruct.[258] It is important to supply adequate amounts of vitamin C to the body every day,[259] and because very little of what you take orally makes it into your bloodstream,[260] this is an important vitamin to take daily at RDA recommended amounts. The most well-known example of a deficiency of vitamin C is scurvy (the old seafarer disease).[261] There is no need to exceed RDA recommendations because high levels of vitamin C can adversely affect the kidneys.[262] Many one-a-day multivitamins will more than meet all your vitamin needs, even for vitamins B_{12}, C, and D.

Your body also needs a variety of minerals. Older folks have an unhealthy depletion of sodium as they age,[263] which can also accelerate diabetic complications.[264] One great source of minerals is naturally enriched salts like sea, Celtic, Himalayan, or lava salts. Salt used to be blamed for hypertension,[265] but we now know that hypertension is related to impairment in circulation[266] and meat consumption.[267] Once we clean and clear the blood and its pathways in otherwise healthy people, salt sensitivity goes away. As soon as your blood pressure and sugar levels start to normalize on the Wash Cycle Diet, consume normal amounts of mineral heavy salts.[268] Look for mineral salts with an orange or darker tint with a four to one concentration of salt to minerals. Mix mineral salts from different regions of the world.[269] The complexity and variety of natural matter found in these mineral salts will provide a good portion of the electrolytes and minerals your body requires.

Your body also needs a small amount of naturally derived elements that come from decomposed organic matter. Fulvic minerals contain Fulvic and humic acids that provide benefits to health and the body including boosting the immune system, decreasing inflammation, improving brain function, reducing fatigue, and aiding iron absorption. There are many sources for fulvic minerals buit my preference is Shilajit, a compound with high amounts of natural organic matter like humic and fulvic acid, bonded to a large mix of different minerals like iron, zinc, magnesium, and potassium, as well as other compounds that have spent years developing complexity, in a very bio-available form.[270] This mineral extract is sometimes called rock juice, the sweat of mountains or mountain ooze,[271] and has been known for its healing qualities for centuries.[272] Shilajit does taste awful, but a 250mg dose once or twice a month is easy to tolerate.

As high blood fat and cholesterol levels increase, most doctors prescribe statins (Zocor®, Lipitor®, Crestor®), which have been found to be effective at reducing LDL "bad" cholesterol.[273] Millions of people take statins. As blood sugar levels in diabetics start to uncontrollably spike, doctors may also prescribe metformin (Fortamet®, Glucophage®, Riomet®), which have been found to be effective at reducing blood glucose levels. Indian gooseberry (Amla) powder (seed, fruit, and leaf) has also been shown to be effective at reducing cholesterol levels *without* any appreciable side effects.[274] Amla is an ancient medicinal tropical fruit[275] with many touted health benefits.[276] Amla contains many different active plant compounds and a variety of phenolic acids. In one study, a teaspoon of powdered Amla given to participants once daily after breakfast for 21 days significantly decreased total cholesterol and triglyceride values at 8, 15, and 21 days. Amla also appreciably increased HDL cholesterol in some diabetics.[277] Moringa plant powder has similarly helpful effects for diabetics.[278] Moringa also has powerful plant compounds[279] and phenolic acids.[280] Moringa will inhibit the absorption of glucose, fat, and cholesterol in the intestines and liver, and increase insulin sensitivity. In one study, the use of Moringa reduced the blood sugar spike in diabetics at various intervals after a meal.[281]

Amla and Moringa are not replacements for those taking statins and metformin, but what you can do is take Amla and Moringa along with your prescriptions, and once the Wash Cycle Diet normalizes your triglyceride (TG), total cholesterol (TC), and blood glucose levels, you can talk to your doctor about getting off statins and metformin, while you continue with Amla and Moringa as a preventative supplement.

Quercetin, a well-studied plant compound found in larger quantities in coriander/cilantro or yellow onion, promotes “insulin sensitization by stimulating pancreatic β-cell proliferation”.[282] Quercetin has also been shown to lower blood pressure. In a randomized, double-blind, placebo-controlled, crossover study performed with human patients with stage 1 hypertension, administration of high-dose Quercetin led to significant decreases in systolic, diastolic, and mean arterial pressure.[283] Garlic and onion also contain an active ingredient called N-acetylcysteine (also known as N-acetyl-cysteine, NAC), a precursor to the antioxidant glutathione (GSH),[284] with proven cardio-protective properties. Over a period of three months, studies have shown that consumption of black (aged) garlic is quite effective at lowering blood pressure.[285]

Turmeric contains a bioactive molecule called curcumin. Curcumin works like the anti-diabetic drug Thiazolidinedione®, which has been proven effective in the regulation of high fat and sugar blood levels. Curcumin inhibits reactive oxygen species (ROS), reducing inflammatory factors and pathways which cause oxidative damage.[286] Look for piperine-laced (pepper) and/or phytosomal (fat absorbed) curcumin to increase absorption.

Similarly, catechins, found in green teas, can help significantly reduce body weight and fat levels after sustained three months use in higher doses. Studies have shown that cardiovascular disease-associated mortality was greatly reduced in older adults consuming five or more cups of green tea every day. An active ingredient in green tea is epigallocatechin gallate (EGCG). Studies have shown that EGCG up-regulates the mediator Nrf_2 which induces the expression of antioxidants and signals healing in the body. In turn, there is a lower expression of C-reactive protein (CRP) and interleukin-6 (IL-6), both being reliable markers for inflammation. Japanese Sencha has high levels of ECGC. If you decide to brew the tea, do not brew for more than a few minutes at lower temperatures.[287] Catechins transport poorly across the intestinal lining, so a phytosomal green tea laced with a small dose of piperine[288] can be taken in pill form during the wash cycle.[289] Brewed green tea is good for long term use, but to help with weight loss during the Wash Cycle Diet, use the phytosomal green tea pill.

One of the byproducts of animal-based diets and cooking, especially frying and open flame, is the generation of MRPs (maillard reaction products like Advanced Glycation End Products [AGEs] and Heterocyclic Amines [HCAs]).[290] Resveratrol is a strong antioxidant that can help to neutralize these peroxides,[291] and is found in high quantity in grape skins. Black cumin (nagella sativa or black cumin seed) is another plant containing a phenolic compound called thymoquinone,[292] which has been shown to protect against oxidative stress, inflammation, and insulin resistance resulting from obesity in mice.[293] Look for oils of this plant that claim to have 3 to 5% Thymoquinone. One last powerful plant compound is sulforaphane, a potent activator of cellular defense against oxidative stress.[294] Broccoli sprouts, *when chewed up*, make sulforaphane.[295] Sulforaphane is a potent plant compound that brings back the balance lost during aging in systems of your body.[296] The compound actively fights osteoporosis by reversing bone resorption.[297]

There are also several other polyphenols found in plants that can offer protection against depression (saffron),[298] certain cancers, and disease.[299] To date, some eight thousand polyphenols have been identified.[300] We have just started to scratch the surface in understanding the power of plants in improving longevity. Unfortunately, there is still a good deal of misinformation out there. For example, you should be skeptical of any claims about how something that is clearly *not* good for you, such as alcohol, suddenly has redeeming qualities because it contains traces of some plant compound. My favorite is that "antioxidants" in wine are a good reason for you to drink wine. The truth is that a few fresh berries or a teaspoon of cocoa powder or carob powder has twenty times the antioxidants found in a glass of wine.[301] These claims are intended to *enable* you to continue to consume something that is clearly bad for you as you age.

DHA AND EPA

As we age, our brains shrink and we lose much of our brain size.[302] We can slow this process down by increasing the availability of a couple of very specific fats.[303] The Wash Cycle Diet uses raw plant-based omega-rich fats to meet all of our body's needs with nuts, seeds, nut butter, and plant milk.[304] Your liver is also very efficient at turning carbohydrates into fat. But there are two very specific fats that the body has a hard time acquiring and producing: DHA (docosahexaenoic acid) and EPA (eicosapentaenoic acid). DHA and EPA are long-chain fatty acids that have extra kinks that make them more fluid.[305] Our brain has high levels of DHA and we need to make sure that the brain receives as much DHA as it needs to reduce shrinking and calcification as we get older.[306] EPA is also a very fluid fat that acts to improve circulatory function. Healthy endothelial cells line our blood pathways and allow for the transport of nutrients and waste. Although our digestive systems will destroy or convert most of the things we consume, an EPA/DHA supplement can help.[307] The amount you need comes in a small capsule or by the teaspoon. You can either take an algae-based or fish-based DHA/EPA-rich oil.[308] Reputable supplement companies have safeguards to eliminate any toxins from their DHA/EPA fish oil-based supplements.

PROBIOTICS/FERMENTED FOODS

Studies have found positive results when the right types of probiotics are taken,[309] and it is claimed that you can even use good bacteria to help fight degeneration and chronic disease.[310] Fermented foods are excellent sources of "good" microbes. As a part of the Wash Cycle Diet, feel free to consume fermented vegetables[311] or nut-based cheeses. I do not cover fermenting deeply in this book, but YouTube has many videos on how to ferment vegetables and nuts. There are also many recipe books on the subject. There is a fermented sprout drink that was championed by Ms. Wigmore called Rejuvelac.[312] You can find a link to how to make this drink on our website (rawrevolution.biz).

This is a good spot to also talk about antibiotics. Broad-spectrum antibiotics destroy good and bad bacteria indiscriminately.[313] Antibiotics "influence the function of the immune system, our ability to resist infection, and our capacity for processing food."[314] Antibiotics promote weight gain,[315] early life exposure to antibiotics is related to later metabolic disease,[316] and killing your gut bacteria with antibiotics can have major repercussions on your health.[317] Try to avoid indiscriminate antibiotic use as an aging diabetic because it is much harder to replenish good bacteria in your body after a course of bacterial genocide in your gut. If you do need to take antibiotics, during and for a while after you have completed your course of antibiotics, eat fermented foods or nut cheeses to try and bring back some of the good bacteria you killed off. It is very important to make sure you keep your gut bacteria plentiful and healthy.

These extra tweaks, along with diet modification, will keep you well-regulated and healthy over the coming years. Most importantly, listen to your body, especially when it's trying to tell you something. Subtle uncontrollable twitches, joint pain, neck pain, headaches, or depression are complaints being lodged by your body. On the other hand, happiness, joy, extra energy, and waking up refreshed in the morning pain free means your body is happy and satisfied.

---

[202]Schoeller DA. Changes in total body water with age. Am J ClinNutr. 1989

Nov;50(5 Suppl):1176-81; discussion 1231-5. doi: 10.1093/ajcn/50.5.1176. PMID: 2683726 DOI: 10.1093/ajcn/50.5.1176.

[203]Cowen LE, Hodak SP, VerbalisJG.Age-associated abnormalities of water homeostasis. *EndocrinolMetabClin North Am.* 2013;42(2):349-70.

[204]Begg, DP. Disturbances of thirst and fluid balance associated with aging. PhysiolBehav. 2017 Sep 1;178:28-34. doi: 10.1016/j.physbeh.2017.03.003. Epub 2017 Mar 4. Review.

[205]Hooper L, Bunn D, Jimoh FO, Fairweather-Tait SJ.Water-loss dehydrationMech Ageing Dev. 2014 Mar-Apr;136-137:50-8. doi: 10.1016/j.mad.2013.11.009. Epub 2013 Dec 9. Review.

[206]Stachenfeld NS, Leone CA, Mitchell ES, Freese E, Harkness L. Water intake reverses dehydration PhysiolBehav. 2018 Mar 1;185:103-111. doi: 10.1016/j.physbeh.2017.12.028. Epub 2017 Dec 23.

[207]Cowen LE, Hodak SP, VerbalisJG.Age-associated abnormalities of water homeostasis. *EndocrinolMetabClin North Am.* 2013;42(2):349-70.

[208]Cowen LE, Hodak SP, VerbalisJG.Age-Associated Abnormalities of Water Homeostasis. *Endocrinology and metabolism clinics of North America.* 2013;42(2):349-370. doi:10.1016/j.ecl.2013.02.005.

[209]Sagar PS, Zhang J, Luciuk M, Mannix C, Wong ATY, Rangan GK. Increased water intake reduces long-term renal and cardiovascular disease progression in experimental polycystic kidney disease. *PLoS One.* 2019;14(1):e0209186. Published 2019 Jan 2. doi:10.1371/journal.pone.0209186

[210] Hamasaki H. Daily physical activity and type 2 diabetes: A review. *World J Diabetes.* 2016;7(12):243–251. doi:10.4239/wjd.v7.i12.243

[211]Nilsson MI, Tarnopolsky MA. Mitochondria and Aging-The Role of Exercise as a Countermeasure. *Biology (Basel).* 2019;8(2):40. Published 2019 May 11. doi:10.3390/biology8020040

[212] Reynolds AN, Venn BJ.The Timing of Activity after Eating Affects the Glycaemic Response of Healthy Adults: A Randomised Controlled Trial. *Nutrients.* 2018;10(11):1743. Published 2018 Nov 13. doi:10.3390/nu10111743

[213] Your lungs and exercise. *Breathe (Sheff).* 2016;12(1):97–100. doi:10.1183/20734

[214] Genuis SJ, Beesoon S, Birkholz D. Biomonitoring and Elimination of Perfluorinated Compounds and Polychlorinated Biphenyls through Perspiration: Blood, Urine, and Sweat Study. *ISRN Toxicol.* 2013;2013:483832. Published 2013 Sep 3. doi:10.1155/2013/483832

[215] He C, Sumpter R Jr, Levine B. Exercise induces autophagy in peripheral tissues and in the brain. *Autophagy.* 2012;8(10):1548–1551. doi:10.4161/auto.21327

[216]Hussain J, Cohen M. Clinical Effects of Regular Dry Sauna Bathing: A Systematic Review. *Evid Based Complement Alternat Med.* 2018;2018:1857413. Published 2018 Apr 24. doi:10.1155/2018/1857413

[217]Laukkanen T, Kunutsor SK, Khan H, Willeit P, Zaccardi F, Laukkanen JA. Sauna bathing is associated with reduced cardiovascular mortality and improves risk prediction in men and women: a prospective cohort study. *BMC Med.* 2018;16(1):219. Published 2018 Nov 29. doi:10.1186/s12916-018-1198-0

[218] Sawka MN, Montain SJ. Fluid and electrolyte supplementation for exercise heat stress. Am J Clin Nutr. 2000 Aug;72(2 Suppl):564S-72S. doi: 10.1093/ajcn/72.2.564S. Review.

[219]Hussain J, Cohen M. Clinical Effects of Regular Dry Sauna Bathing: A Systematic Review. *Evid Based Complement Alternat Med.* 2018;2018:1857413. Published 2018 Apr 24. doi:10.1155/2018/1857413

[220] Schroeder AM, Colwell CS. How to fix a broken clock. *Trends Pharmacol Sci.* 2013;34(11):605–619. doi:10.1016/j.tips.2013.09.002

[221] Zielinski MR, McKenna JT, McCarley RW. Functions and Mechanisms of Sleep. *AIMS Neurosci.* 2016;3(1):67–104. doi:10.3934/Neuroscience.2016.1.67

[222] Hardeland R. Neurobiology, pathophysiology, and treatment of melatonin deficiency and dysfunction. *Scientific World Journal.* 2012;2012:640389. doi:10.1100/2012/640389

[223] Seifalian A, Hart A. Circadian Rhythms: Will It Revolutionise the Management of Diseases?. *J Lifestyle Med.* 2019;9(1):1–11. doi:10.15280/jlm.2019.9.1.1

[224] Vercruysse P, Vieau D, Blum D, Petersén Å, Dupuis L. Hypothalamic Alterations in Neurodegenerative Diseases and Their Relation to Abnormal Energy Metabolism. *Front Mol Neurosci.* 2018;11:2. Published 2018 Jan 19.

doi:10.3389/fnmol.2018.00002

[225] Zhou L, Gao Q, Nie M, et al. Degeneration and energy shortage in the suprachiasmatic nucleus underlies the circadian rhythm disturbance in $ApoE^{-/-}$ mice: implications for Alzheimer's disease. *Sci Rep*. 2016;6:36335. Published 2016 Nov 8. doi:10.1038/srep36335

[226] Arora T, Taheri S. Sleep Optimization and Diabetes Control: A Review of the Literature. *Diabetes Ther*. 2015;6(4):425–468. doi:10.1007/s13300-015-0141-z

[227] Potter GD, Skene DJ, Arendt J, Cade JE, Grant PJ, Hardie LJ. Circadian Rhythm and Sleep Disruption: Causes, Metabolic Consequences, and Countermeasures. *Endocr Rev*. 2016;37(6):584–608. doi:10.1210/er.2016-1083

[228]Knutson KL, Ryden AM, Mander BA, Van Cauter E. Role of sleep duration and quality in the risk and severity of type 2 diabetes mellitus. Arch Intern Med. 2006;166(16):1768–1774. doi: 10.1001/archinte.166.16.1768.

[229] Xie L, Kang H, Xu Q, et al. Sleep drives metabolite clearance from the adult brain. *Science*. 2013;342(6156):373–377. doi:10.1126/science.1241224

[230] McMillan A, Morrell MJ. Sleep disordered breathing at the extremes of age: the elderly. *Breathe (Sheff)*. 2016;12(1):50–60. doi:10.1183/20734735.003216

[231] Phan TX, Malkani RG. Sleep and circadian rhythm disruption and stress intersect in Alzheimer's disease. *Neurobiol Stress*. 2018;10:100133. Published 2018 Oct 17. doi:10.1016/j.ynstr.2018.10.001

[232] Patel D, Steinberg J, Patel P. Insomnia in the Elderly: A Review. *J Clin Sleep Med*. 2018;14(6):1017–1024. Published 2018 Jun 15. doi:10.5664/jcsm.7172

[233] Harding EC, Franks NP, Wisden W. The Temperature Dependence of Sleep. *Front Neurosci*. 2019;13:336. Published 2019 Apr 24. doi:10.3389/fnins.2019.00336

[234] Bonomini F, Borsani E, Favero G, Rodella LF, Rezzani R. Dietary Melatonin Supplementation Could Be a Promising Preventing/Therapeutic Approach for a Variety of Liver Diseases. *Nutrients*. 2018;10(9):1135. Published 2018 Aug 21. doi:10.3390/nu10091135

[235] Chellan P, Sadler PJ. The elements of life and medicines. *Philos Trans A Math Phys Eng Sci*. 2015;373(2037):20140182. doi:10.1098/rsta.2014.0182

[236] Chen F, et al. Association Among Dietary Supplement Use, Nutrient Intake, and Mortality Among U.S. Adults: A Cohort Study. Ann Intern Med. 2019 May 7;170(9):604-613. doi: 10.7326/M18-2478. Epub 2019 Apr 9.

[237] Bahadoran Z, Mirmiran P, Azizi F. Dietary polyphenols as potential nutraceuticals in management of diabetes: a review. *J Diabetes Metab Disord*. 2013;12(1):43. Published 2013 Aug 13. doi:10.1186/2251-6581-12-43

[238]Ames BN. Low micronutrient intake may accelerate the degenerative diseases of aging through allocation of scarce micronutrients by triage. *Proc Natl AcadSci U S A*. 2006;103(47):17589–17594. doi:10.1073/pnas.0608757103

[239] Maggini S, Pierre A, Calder PC. Immune Function and Micronutrient Requirements Change over the Life Course. *Nutrients*. 2018;10(10):1531. Published 2018 Oct 17. doi:10.3390/nu10101531

[240] Krishnaswamy K, Gayathri R. Nature's bountiful gift to humankind: Vegetables & fruits & their role in cardiovascular disease & diabetes. *Indian J Med Res*. 2018;148(5):569–595. doi:10.4103/ijmr.IJMR_1780_18

[241] National Research Council (US) Subcommittee on the Tenth Edition of the Recommended Dietary Allowances. Recommended Dietary Allowances: 10th Edition. Washington (DC): National Academies Press (US); 1989. Available from: https://www.ncbi.nlm.nih.gov/books/NBK234932/ doi: 10.17226/1349

[242]Kift R, Rhodes LE, Farrar MD, Webb AR. Is Sunlight Exposure Enough to Avoid Wintertime Vitamin D Deficiency in United Kingdom Population Groups?. *Int J Environ Res Public Health*. 2018;15(8):1624. Published 2018 Aug 1. doi:10.3390/ijerph15081624

[243]Chen L, Dong Y, Bhagatwala J, Raed A, Huang Y, Zhu H. Effects of Vitamin D3 Supplementation on Epigenetic Aging in Overweight and Obese African Americans With Suboptimal Vitamin D Status: A Randomized Clinical Trial.JGerontol A BiolSci Med Sci. 2019 Jan 1;74(1):91-98. doi: 10.1093/gerona/gly223.

[244] Ghareghani M, Reiter RJ, Zibara K, Farhadi N. Latitude, Vitamin D, Melatonin, and Gut Microbiota Act in Concert to Initiate Multiple Sclerosis: A New Mechanistic Pathway. *Front Immunol*. 2018;9:2484. Published 2018 Oct

30. doi:10.3389/fimmu.2018.02484

[245] Going CC, Alexandrova L, Lau K, Yeh CY, Feldman D, Pitteri SJ. Vitamin D supplementation decreases serum 27-hydroxycholesterol in a pilot breast cancer trial. *Breast Cancer Res Treat.* 2018;167(3):797–802. doi:10.1007/s10549-017-4562-4

[246]Zadka K, Pałkowska-Goździk E, Rosołowska-HuszczD.The State of Knowledge about Nutrition Sources of Vitamin D, Its Role in the Human Body, and Necessity of Supplementation among Parents in Central Poland. *Int J Environ Res Public Health.* 2018;15(7):1489. Published 2018 Jul 14. doi:10.3390/ijerph15071489

[247]Zhou Z, Zhou R, Zhang Z, Li K. The Association Between Vitamin D Status, Vitamin D Supplementation, Sunlight Exposure, and Parkinson's Disease: A Systematic Review and Meta-Analysis. *Med SciMonit.* 2019;25:666–674. Published 2019 Jan 23. doi:10.12659/MSM.912840

[248]Sadat-Ali M, Al-Anii FM, Al-Turki HA, AlBadran AA, AlShammari SM. Maintenance Dose of Vitamin D: How Much Is Enough?. *J Bone Metab.* 2018;25(3):161–164. doi:10.11005/jbm.2018.25.3.161

[249]Letavernier E, Daudon M. Vitamin D, Hypercalciuria and Kidney Stones. *Nutrients.* 2018;10(3):366. Published 2018 Mar 17. doi:10.3390/nu10030366

[250]Li K, Wang XF, Li DY, et al. The good, the bad, and the ugly of calcium supplementation: a review of calcium intake on human health. *ClinInterv Aging.* 2018;13:2443–2452. Published 2018 Nov 28. doi:10.2147/CIA.S157523

[251]Chandra P, Wolfenden LL, Ziegler TR, et al. Treatment of vitamin D deficiency with UV light in patients with malabsorption syndromes: a case series. *PhotodermatolPhotoimmunolPhotomed.* 2007;23(5):179–185. doi:10.1111/j.1600-0781.2007.00302.x

[252] van Ballegooijen AJ, Pilz S, Tomaschitz A, Grübler MR, Verheyen N. The Synergistic Interplay between Vitamins D and K for Bone and Cardiovascular Health: A Narrative Review. *Int J Endocrinol.* 2017;2017:7454376. doi:10.1155/2017/7454376

[253] van de Lagemaat EE, de Groot LCPGM, van den Heuvel EGHM. Vitamin B_{12} in Relation to Oxidative Stress: A Systematic Review. *Nutrients.* 2019;11(2):482. Published 2019 Feb 25. doi:10.3390/nu11020482

[254] Wolffenbuttel BHR, Wouters HJCM, Heiner-Fokkema MR, van der Klauw MM. The Many Faces of Cobalamin (Vitamin B_{12}) Deficiency. *Mayo Clin Proc Innov Qual Outcomes*. 2019;3(2):200–214. Published 2019 May 27. doi:10.1016/j.mayocpiqo.2019.03.002

[255] Donaldson MS. Metabolic vitamin B12 status on a mostly raw diet with follow-up using tablets, nutritional yeast, or probiotic supplements. Ann Nutr Metab. 2000;44(5-6):229-34.

[256]McGregor GP, Biesalski HK. Rationale and impact of vitamin C in clinical nutrition.CurrOpinClinNutrMetab Care. 2006 Nov;9(6):697-703. PMID: 17053422 DOI:10.1097/01.mco.0000247478.79779.8f.

[257]Young JI, Züchner S, Wang G. Regulation of the Epigenome by Vitamin C. *Annual review of nutrition*. 2015;35:545-564. doi:10.1146/annurev-nutr-071714-034228.

[258]Lu Y-X, Wu Q-N, Chen D, et al. Pharmacological Ascorbate Suppresses Growth of Gastric Cancer Cells with GLUT1 Overexpression and Enhances the Efficacy of Oxaliplatin Through Redox Modulation. *Theranostics*. 2018;8(5):1312-1326. doi:10.7150/thno.21745.

[259]Vissers MCM, Das AB. Potential Mechanisms of Action for Vitamin C in Cancer: Reviewing the Evidence. *Frontiers in Physiology*. 2018;9:809. doi:10.3389/fphys.2018.00809.

[260]Carr AC, Pullar JM, Bozonet SM, Vissers MCM. Marginal Ascorbate Status (Hypovitaminosis C) Results in an Attenuated Response to Vitamin C Supplementation. *Nutrients*. 2016;8(6):341. doi:10.3390/nu8060341.

[261]Delanghe JR, Langlois MR, De Buyzere ML, et al. Vitamin C deficiency: more than just a nutritional disorder. *Genes & Nutrition*. 2011;6(4):341-346. doi:10.1007/s12263-011-0237-7.

[262]Lin WV, Turin CG, McCormick DW, Haas C, Constantine G. Ascorbic acid-induced oxalate nephropathy: a case report and discussion of pathologic mechanisms. *CEN Case Rep*. ;8(1):67–70. doi:10.1007/s13730-018-0366-6

[263]Filippatos TD, Makri A, Elisaf MS, Liamis G. Hyponatremia in the elderly: challenges and solutions. *ClinInterv Aging*. 2017;12:1957-1965. Published 2017 Nov 14. doi:10.2147/CIA.S138535

[264]Liamis G, Liberopoulos E, Barkas F, Elisaf M. Diabetes mellitus and electrolyte disorders. *World J Clin Cases*. 2014;2(10):488-96.

[265] National Research Council (US) Committee on Diet and Health. Diet and Health: Implications for Reducing Chronic Disease Risk. Washington (DC): National Academies Press (US); 1989. 15, Electrolytes.

[266]Choi HY, Park HC, Ha SK. Salt Sensitivity and Hypertension: A Paradigm Shift from Kidney Malfunction to Vascular Endothelial Dysfunction. *Electrolytes & Blood Pressure : E & BP*. 2015;13(1):7-16. doi:10.5049/EBP.2015.13.1.7.

[267] Oude Griep LM, Seferidi P, Stamler J, et al. Relation of unprocessed, processed red meat and poultry consumption to blood pressure in East Asian and Western adults. *J Hypertens*. 2016;34(9):1721-1729. doi:10.1097/HJH.0000000000001008

[268] Lee BH, Yang AR, Kim MY, McCurdy S, Boisvert WA. Natural sea salt consumption confers protection against hypertension and kidney damage in Dahl salt-sensitive rats [published correction appears in Food Nutr Res. 2017 Mar 20;61(1):1300375]. *Food Nutr Res*. 2016;61(1):1264713. Published 2016 Dec 20. doi:10.1080/16546628.2017.1264713

[269]Ju J, Song JL, Park ES, Do MS, Park KY. Korean solar salts reduce obesity and alter its related markers in diet-induced obese mice. *Nutr Res Pract*. 2016;10(6):629-634.

[270] Mirza MA, Ahmad N, Agarwal SP, Mahmood D, Khalid Anwer M, Iqbal Z. Comparative evaluation of humic substances in oral drug delivery. *Results Pharma Sci*. 2011;1(1):16-26. Published 2011 Jul 12. doi:10.1016/j.rinphs.2011.06.001

[271] Cagno V, Donalisio M, Civra A, Cagliero C, Rubiolo P, Lembo D. In vitro evaluation of the antiviral properties of Shilajit and investigation of its mechanisms of action. *J Ethnopharmacol*. 2015;166:129-134. doi:10.1016/j.jep.2015.03.019

[272] Biswas TK, Pandit S, Mondal S, et al. Clinical evaluation of spermatogenic activity of processed Shilajit in oligospermia. *Andrologia*. 2010;42(1):48-56. doi:10.1111/j.1439-0272.2009.00956.x

[273] Ramkumar, S. Wilson A. (2015). Statins: Review of safety and potential side effects. Heart, Lung and Circulation, 24. Doi:10/1016/j.hic.2015.06.184

[274] Upadya H, et al. A randomized, double blind, placebo controlled,

multicenter clinical trial to assess the efficacy and safety of Emblica officinalis extract in patients with dyslipidemia. *BMC Complement Altern Med.* 2019;19(1):27. Published 2019 Jan 22. doi:10.1186/s12906-019-2430-y

[275] Upadya H, Prabhu S, Prasad A, Subramanian D, Gupta S, Goel A. A randomized, double blind, placebo controlled, multicenter clinical trial to assess the efficacy and safety of Emblica officinalis extract in patients with dyslipidemia. *BMC Complement Altern Med.* 2019;19(1):27. Published 2019 Jan 22. doi:10.1186/s12906-019-2430-y

[276] Tewari R, Kumar V, Sharma HK. Physical and chemical characteristics of different cultivars of Indian gooseberry (*Emblica officinalis*). J Food Sci Technol. 2019 Mar;56(3):1641-1648. doi: 10.1007/s13197-019-03595-y. Epub 2019 Feb 7.

[277] Akhtar MS, et al. Effect of Amla fruit on blood glucose and lipid profile of normal subjects and type 2 diabetic patients. Int J Food Sci Nutr. 2011 Sep;62(6):609-16. doi: 10.3109/09637486.2011.560565. Epub 2011 Apr 18.

[278]Abd Rani NZ, Husain K, Kumolosasi E. *Moringa* Genus: A Review of Phytochemistry and Pharmacology. *Front Pharmacol.* 2018;9:108. Published 2018 Feb 16. doi:10.3389/fphar.2018.00108

[279] Nova E, Redondo-Useros N, Martínez-García RM, Gómez-Martínez S, Díaz-Prieto LE, Marcos A. Potential of *Moringa oleifera* to Improve Glucose Control for the Prevention of Diabetes and Related Metabolic Alterations: A Systematic Review of Animal and Human Studies. *Nutrients.* 2020;12(7):2050. Published 2020 Jul 10. doi:10.3390/nu12072050

[280] Kou X, Li B, Olayanju JB, Drake JM, Chen N. Nutraceutical or Pharmacological Potential of Moringa oleifera Lam. *Nutrients.* 2018;10(3):343. Published 2018 Mar 12. doi:10.3390/nu10030343

[281] Leone A, Bertoli S, Di Lello S, et al. Effect of *Moringa oleifera* Leaf Powder on Postprandial Blood Glucose Response: In Vivo Study on Saharawi People Living in Refugee Camps. *Nutrients.* 2018;10(10):1494. Published 2018 Oct 12. doi:10.3390/nu10101494

[282] Salehi B, Machin L, Monzote L, et al. Therapeutic Potential of Quercetin: New Insights and Perspectives for Human Health. *ACS Omega.* 2020;5(20):11849-11872. Published 2020 May 14.

doi:10.1021/acsomega.0c01818

[283] Salehi B, Machin L, Monzote L, et al. Therapeutic Potential of Quercetin: New Insights and Perspectives for Human Health. *ACS Omega.* 2020;5(20):11849-11872. Published 2020 May 14. doi:10.1021/acsomega.0c01818

[284] Šalamon Š, Kramar B, Marolt TP, Poljšak B, Milisav I. Medical and Dietary Uses of N-Acetylcysteine. *Antioxidants (Basel).* 2019;8(5):111. Published 2019 Apr 28. doi:10.3390/antiox8050111

[285] Matsutomo T. Potential benefits of garlic and other dietary supplements for the management of hypertension. *Exp Ther Med.* 2020;19(2):1479-1484. doi:10.3892/etm.2019.8375

[286] Pivari F, Mingione A, Brasacchio C, Soldati L. Curcumin and Type 2 Diabetes Mellitus: Prevention and Treatment. *Nutrients.* 2019;11(8):1837. Published 2019 Aug 8. doi:10.3390/nu11081837

[287] Saklar S, Ertas E, Ozdemir IS, Karadeniz B. Effects of different brewing conditions on catechin content and sensory acceptance in Turkish green tea infusions. *J Food Sci Technol.* 2015;52(10):6639-6646. doi:10.1007/s13197-015-1746-y

[288] Cai ZY, Li XM, Liang JP, et al. Bioavailability of Tea Catechins and Its Improvement. *Molecules.* 2018;23(9):2346. Published 2018 Sep 13. doi:10.3390/molecules23092346

[289] Belcaro G, Ledda A, Hu S, Cesarone MR, Feragalli B, Dugall M. Greenselect phytosome for borderline metabolic syndrome. *Evid Based Complement Alternat Med.* 2013;2013:869061. doi:10.1155/2013/869061

[290] Cepas V, Collino M, Mayo JC, Sainz RM. Redox Signaling and Advanced Glycation Endproducts (AGEs) in Diet-Related Diseases. *Antioxidants (Basel).* 2020;9(2):142. Published 2020 Feb 6. doi:10.3390/antiox9020142

[291] Bors W, Heller W, Michel C, Saran M. Flavonoids as antioxidants: determination of radical-scavenging efficiencies. *Methods Enzymol.* 1990;186:343-355. doi:10.1016/0076-6879(90)86128-i

[292] Forouzanfar F, Bazzaz BS, Hosseinzadeh H. Black cumin (Nigella sativa)

and its constituent (thymoquinone): a review on antimicrobial effects. *Iran J Basic Med Sci*. 2014;17(12):929-938.

[293] Shen HH, Peterson SJ, Bellner L, et al. Cold-Pressed *Nigella Sativa* Oil Standardized to 3% Thymoquinone Potentiates Omega-3 Protection against Obesity-Induced Oxidative Stress, Inflammation, and Markers of Insulin Resistance Accompanied with Conversion of White to Beige Fat in Mice. *Antioxidants (Basel)*. 2020;9(6):489. Published 2020 Jun 4. doi:10.3390/antiox9060489

[294] Bai Y, Wang X, Zhao S, Ma C, Cui J, Zheng Y. Sulforaphane Protects against Cardiovascular Disease via Nrf2 Activation. *Oxid Med Cell Longev*. 2015;2015:407580. doi:10.1155/2015/407580

[295] Kim JK, Park SU. Current potential health benefits of sulforaphane. *EXCLI J*. 2016;15:571–577. Published 2016 Oct 13. doi:10.17179/excli2016-485

[296] Kubo E, Chhunchha B, Singh P, Sasaki H, Singh DP. Sulforaphane reactivates cellular antioxidant defense by inducing Nrf2/ARE/Prdx6 activity during aging and oxidative stress. *Sci Rep*. 2017;7(1):14130. Published 2017 Oct 26. doi:10.1038/s41598-017-14520-8

[297] Thaler R, Maurizi A, Roschger P, et al. Anabolic and Antiresorptive Modulation of Bone Homeostasis by the Epigenetic Modulator Sulforaphane, a Naturally Occurring Isothiocyanate. *J Biol Chem*. 2016;291(13):6754-6771. doi:10.1074/jbc.M115.678235

[298] Wang Y, Han T, Zhu Y, Zheng CJ, Ming QL, Rahman K, Qin LP. Antidepressant properties of bioactive fractions from the extract of Crocus sativus L. J Nat Med. 2010 Jan;64(1):24-30. doi: 10.1007/s11418-009-0360-6. Epub 2009 Sep 29. PMID: 19787421.

[299] Pandey KB, Rizvi SI. Plant polyphenols as dietary antioxidants in human health and disease. *Oxid Med Cell Longev*. 2009;2(5):270-278. doi:10.4161/oxim.2.5.9498

[300] Cory H, Passarelli S, Szeto J, Tamez M, Mattei J. The Role of Polyphenols in Human Health and Food Systems: A Mini-Review. *Front Nutr*. 2018;5:87. Published 2018 Sep 21. doi:10.3389/fnut.2018.00087

[301] Rothwell, JA. et al., Phenol-Explorer 3.0: a major update of the Phenol-

Explorer database to incorporate data on the effects of food processing on polyphenol content, *Database*, Volume 2013, 2013, bat070, https://doi.org/10.1093/database/bat070

[302] Peters R. Ageing and the brain. *Postgrad Med J.* 2006;82(964):84–88. doi:10.1136/pgmj.2005.036665

[303] Chianese R, Coccurello R, Viggiano A, et al. Impact of Dietary Fats on Brain Functions. *Curr Neuropharmacol.* 2018;16(7):1059–1085. doi:10.2174/1570159X15666171017102547

[304] Saini RK, Keum YS. Omega-3 and omega-6 polyunsaturated fatty acids: Dietary sources, metabolism Life Sci. 2018 Jun 15;203:255-267. doi: 10.1016/j.lfs.2018.04.049. Epub 2018 Apr 30. Review.

[305] Bradbury J. Docosahexaenoic acid (DHA): an ancient nutrient for the modern human brain. *Nutrients.* 2011;3(5):529–554. doi:10.3390/nu3050529

[306] Derbyshire E. Brain Health across the Lifespan: A Systematic Review on the Role of Omega-3 Fatty Acid Supplements. *Nutrients.* 2018;10(8):1094. Published 2018 Aug 15. doi:10.3390/nu10081094

[307] Preston Mason R. New Insights into Mechanisms of Action for Omega-3 Fatty Acids in Atherothrombotic Cardiovascular Disease. *Curr Atheroscler Rep.* 2019;21(1):2. Published 2019 Jan 12. doi:10.1007/s11883-019-0762-1

[308]Lenihan-Geels G, Bishop KS, Ferguson LR.Alternative Sources of Omega-3 Fats: Can We Find a Sustainable Substitute for Fish? *Nutrients.* 2013;5(4):1301-1315. doi:10.3390/nu5041301.

[309]Markowiak P, Śliżewska K. Effects of Probiotics, Prebiotics, and Synbiotics on Human Health. *Nutrients.* 2017;9(9):1021. doi:10.3390/nu9091021.

[310]Cerdó T, Ruíz A, Suárez A, Campoy C. Probiotic, Prebiotic, and Brain Development. *Nutrients.* 2017;9(11):1247. doi:10.3390/nu9111247.

[311] Rezac S, Kok CR, Heermann M, Hutkins R. Fermented Foods as a Dietary Source of Live Organisms. *Front Microbiol.* 2018;9:1785. Published 2018 Aug 24. doi:10.3389/fmicb.2018.01785

[312]Wigmore, A. Recipes for Longer Life, Avery (1982).

[313]Gillings MR, Paulsen IT, Tetu SG. Ecology and Evolution of the Human

Microbiota: Fire, Farming and Antibiotics. Iredell J, Partridge S, eds. *Genes*. 2015;6(3):841-857. doi:10.3390/genes6030841.

[314]Langdon A, Crook N, Dantas G. The effects of antibiotics on the microbiome throughout development and alternative approaches for therapeutic modulation. *Genome Medicine*. 2016;8:39. doi:10.1186/s13073-016-0294-z.

[315]Liou AP, TurnbaughPJ. Antibiotic Exposure Promotes Fat Gain. *Cell metabolism*. 2012;16(4):408-410. doi:10.1016/j.cmet.2012.09.009.

[316]Li J, Yang K, Ju T, et al. Early life antibiotic exposure affects pancreatic islet development and metabolic regulation. *Scientific Reports*. 2017;7:41778. doi:10.1038/srep41778.

[317]Fujisaka S, Ussar S, Clish C, et al. Antibiotic effects on gut microbiota and metabolism are host dependent. *The Journal of Clinical Investigation*. 2016;126(12):4430-4443. doi:10.1172/JCI86674.

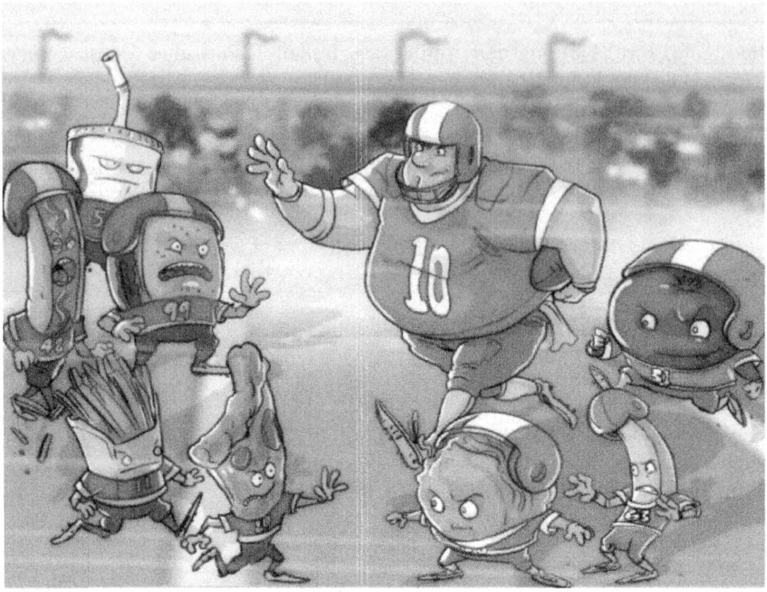

CHAPTER 6

CENTENARIAN

Let's recap what we've learned so far. The goal of this book is to reverse Metabolic Syndrome (MetS), but the implications of the recommendations here are far-reaching.[318] Unless you alter your Western lifestyle, harmful synthetic chemicals will keep damaging your pancreas, liver, and kidneys.[319] Table and liquid sugar, oils, animal fats, and complex proteins will prevent clean-up, keep your arteries rigid, block transport to your cells, inflame your organs, and deteriorate your muscles and bones.[320] Cooking will increase the intake of calories and toxins.[321]

If you are already at the point where you regularly cramp, please take these cramps very seriously. Cramps usually start as flutters in your calves and slowly make their way to your lower abdomen, and/or around your heart, side, chest, and stomach area. If you have constant radiating pain on the heart (left) side of your body that seems to get worse when you indulge in alcohol, caffeine, nicotine, or legal drugs, you need to eliminate or significantly reduce these sources of irritation. If you have memory problems, this is usually a sign of high cholesterol levels.[322] If you have slight weakness or a lack of mobility in your left arm, talk to a doctor. If you find your keys in the refrigerator, you are probably already suffering some level of dementia.

As you implement the Wash Cycle Diet, keep track of your weight, blood fat/sugar levels, and blood pressure regularly. Check your A1c every month. Take note of aches when you wake up, headaches during the day, stiffness around the neck, joint pain in the hips and feet, tingling in the extremities (especially the toes or on the underside of your feet), and difficulty sleeping when you start the cycle so you can see the improvement over the next four months. Pay close attention to your evening and morning blood pressure. Look for pulse spikes and lower oxygen saturation levels.

Strictly adhere to the Wash Cycle Diet for the first four months and maybe even a second four months.[323] If you start to lose too much weight during the first Wash Cycle, by all means, increase your daily feeding window and cooked carbohydrate intake (cook your vegetables or increase legumes consumption), but continue to stay away from sugar, flour, oil, and all animal products. The Wash Cycle Diet has the following features:

► No Processed Cooked Foods: Eat all the raw fruits, vegetables, nuts and seeds, and cooked beans you like and stay away from meat, especially ground meats, dairy products, eggs, oil, frying, or ultra-processed ingredients like flour, sugar, and milk.

► Organic: Food sources must be as free of synthetic chemicals as possible.

► Intermittent fasting: Reduce eating to one meal a day or, at most, to the middle four hours of the day.

► Water: Drink half your weight in ounces of water every day but stop drinking about four hours before bed.

► Micronutrient Supplementation: Take regular doses of B/C/D vitamins, adequate amounts of sea salt, phenolic compounds, and minerals.

► Shake and Bake: Walk 30 minutes every day or do other low-impact exercises to improve circulation like yoga; sit in a sauna for 15 minutes of heat therapy twice a week, and try to get 20 minutes of direct sunlight every day.

► Sleep: Get seven to nine hours of sleep every night in a dark, climate-controlled, and quiet room; take melatonin and read if you are unable to quiet your mind.

A diet filled with raw plants, high in cleaning compounds (onions, garlic, and B and C vitamins), along with mineral salts, sun, exercise, heat, and sleep will slowly clear up oxidation and calcification and stop muscle and bone loss. You will reverse inflammation and restore balance. Even the progression of late-life onset cognitive decline can be dampened with strict adherence to a Wash Cycle lifestyle. Once you are at optimal metabolism, if you start to fall off the wagon, Western foods will usually have a noticeable and immediate adverse response, and the pain and discomfort will quickly return in as little as two to three days.[324]

When I fall off the wagon, it is obvious to me. Heartburn comes back, especially if I consumed alcohol. I usually get a headache or joint pain. I start to feel tired and depressed, with a foggy brain or some dullness. Finally, my blood pressure spikes.

I usually tend to fall off the wagon on weekends because my family will want to go to restaurants, or we order pizza, everyone wants ice cream, or friends come over for drinks. You will feel the pressure to indulge to be social. If you do succumb to the pressure, like I do on occasion, you will only have a small window to get back on the wagon before the addictive powers of a Western diet take hold. A very important tip when you do fall off the wagon is to mix the bad foods with a whole bunch of good raw foods, which will reduce the cumulative negative effect of the fall off the wagon.[325] The increased fiber[326] and antioxidants work as a sort of antidote against the toxins and a binder that prevents absorption of quite a bit of the super dense foods.[327]

Let me end by saying that The Wash Cycle Diet is not meant for young and vibrant individuals who desire to live the healthiest and cleanest life possible at a young age. In fact, such a diet may not be as healthy as one might think for a young person because young people need a dense and nutrient-packed diet for growth and development. The Wash Cycle Diet is for folks in the last third of their life, where extra sugars, proteins, and fat are no longer needed, well after the body is done growing, and when the body needs to take a protective and defensive posture. The Wash Cycle Diet is meant to keep an aging body healthy and pain-free so the person can become a centenarian without medical complications, blindness, loss of hearing, or lack of mobility.[328]

In 1950, there were 3,000 American centenarians, in 2014 there were 72,000, and it is estimated that by 2050 there might be one million centenarians. Let's get there together while still being independent and mobile.[329] Caloric restriction, intermittent fasting, supplementation, and your new healthy lifestyle will get you there by getting rid of the built-up oxidation and calcification inside you and keeping your metabolism as healthy and efficient as possible.[330]

---

[318]Donaldson MS. Nutrition and cancer: a review of the evidence for an anti-cancer diet. *Nutr J.* 2004;3:19. Published 2004 Oct 20. doi:10.1186/1475-2891-3-19

[319]Lee YM, Jacobs DR Jr, Lee DH. Persistent Organic Pollutants and Type 2 Diabetes: A Critical Review of Review Articles. *Front Endocrinol (Lausanne)*. 2018;9:712. Published 2018 Nov 27. doi:10.3389/fendo.2018.00712

[320] Barr AJ. The biochemical basis of disease. *Essays Biochem*. 2018;62(5):619–642. Published 2018 Dec 2. doi:10.1042/EBC20170054

[321] Gray JI, Morton ID. Some toxic compounds produced in food by cooking and processing. J Hum Nutr. 1981 Feb;35(1):5-23. Review.

[322] Schreurs BG. The effects of cholesterol on learning and memory. *Neurosci Biobehav Rev*. 2010;34(8):1366–1379. doi:10.1016/j.neubiorev.2010.04.010

[323]Clinton CM, O'Brien S, Law J, Renier CM, Wendt MR. Whole-foods, plant-based diet alleviates the symptoms of osteoarthritis. *Arthritis*. 2015;2015:708152. doi:10.1155/2015/708152

[324]Attuquayefio T, Stevenson RJ, Oaten MJ, Francis HM. A four-day Western-style dietary intervention causes reductions in hippocampal-dependent learning and memory and interoceptive sensitivity. *PLoS One*. 2017;12(2):e0172645. Published 2017 Feb 23. doi:10.1371/journal.pone.0172645

[325] Cilla A, Alegría A, Attanzio A, Garcia-Llatas G, Tesoriere L, Livrea MA. Dietary phytochemicals in the protection against oxysterol-induced damage. Chem Phys Lipids. 2017 Oct;207(Pt B):192-205. doi: 10.1016/j.chemphyslip.2017.03.001. Epub 2017 Mar 4. Review.

[326] Whisner CM, Angadi SS, Weltman NY, et al. Effects of Low-Fat and High-Fat Meals, with and without Dietary Fiber, on Postprandial Endothelial Function, Triglyceridemia, and Glycemia in Adolescents. *Nutrients*. 2019;11(11):2626. Published 2019 Nov 2. doi:10.3390/nu11112626

[327] Li Z, Wong A, Henning SM, Zhang Y, Jones A, Zerlin A, Thames G, Bowerman S, Tseng CH, Heber D. Hass avocado modulates postprandial vascular reactivity and postprandial inflammatory responses to a hamburger meal in healthy volunteers. Food Funct. 2013 Feb 26;4(3):384-91. doi: 10.1039/c2fo30226h.

[328] Toumpanakis A, Turnbull T, Alba-Barba I. Effectiveness of plant-based diets in promoting well-being in the management of type 2 diabetes: a systematic review. *BMJ Open Diabetes Res Care*. 2018;6(1):e000534. Published 2018 Oct 30. doi:10.1136/bmjdrc-2018-000534

[329] Crimmins EM. Lifespan and Healthspan: Past, Present, and Promise. *Gerontologist.* 2015;55(6):901–911. doi:10.1093/geront/gnv130

[330] TusoPJ, Ismail MH, Ha BP, Bartolotto C. Nutritional Update for Physicians: Plant-Based Diets. *The Permanente Journal.* 2013;17(2):61-66. doi:10.7812/TPP/12-085.

Made in the USA
Monee, IL
04 November 2026

67385830R10075